MW00425382

Acknowledgements

Lucy Pitt and The Pharmacy Show

IPS Specials

Gary Paragpuri, Jennifer Richardson & Chemist and Druggist

Richard Thomas

Carolyn Scott

Pharmacy Podcast

Health Sphere

Pharmacy Forum and Locum Voice

@RxSchoolProblems

@PharmacyProbs

Pharmfinders

Richard Daniszewski

Bradford Association of Pharmacy Students and British Pharmaceutical Students Association

Mike Holden

@pillmanuk

Royal Pharmaceutical Society and The Pharmaceutical Journal

@bookapharmacist

Foreword by Jonathan Mason

Thanks to the wonderful world of social media, Mr Dispenser and I have got to know each other, initially virtually through the Twittersphere, but more recently face-to-face. The wonderful thing about Twitter is that it brings people together from around the World. Mr Dispenser has used social media to engage with pharmacists both in the UK and abroad to compile a wonderfully eclectic collection of anecdotes illustrating the varied, the weird, and the sometimes downright exciting lives of community pharmacists as they go about their day-to-day work, healing the sick, and doing miracles, such as dispensing a twenty item prescription in five minutes flat.

Anyone who has ever worked in a pharmacy will recognise many of the situations faced by their colleagues up and down the country, as well as overseas. We may live and work in different places, but pharmacists, patients, doctors and doctors' receptionists are the same the World over. Which pharmacist hasn't been faced with trying to work out what drug the patient is talking about from their mangled pronunciation, such as Candy Statton (Candesartan), and 'kinky' tablets (Gingko Biloba)? And it's clear that it's not just patients who come up with wonderful new ways of pronouncing drug names: dispensers and pharmacists can be just as bad, particular favourites of mine being Neelm's examples of their dispenser referring to Lamborghini (lamotrigine), Toblerone (tibolone) and "Am-I-triptyline?" ("I don't know, are you?!").

Pharmacists and dispensers the world over will recognise the olfactory pleasures of some of the medicines we dispense. Who doesn't love the smell of Relifex? As well as the rather less enjoyable smells that sometimes assaults our noses: "smells like a chair in an old folk's home" will be recognised, by anyone who's ever dispensed it, as a wonderful description of bendroflumethiazide. Also, we have all had to deal with the aftermath of spilling gloopy liquid medicines.

This compilation provides an insight into the small thrills we experience every day. The joy of being able to drink a hot beverage; the thrill of being rude to customers without their realising it.

This book will be a joy to all who read it. It is a useful guide for new pharmacists about to embark on their careers: these are the things you will be faced with on a daily basis. It is a wonderful read for those of us who have been around for a while – a time to reflect and reminisce.

I was pleased to be able to provide a few anecdotes of my own to Mr Dispenser's wonderful compilation, and I was both honoured and humbled when I received a direct message, via Twitter, from Mr Dispenser asking me to write the foreword for his book. Some of the proceeds will be going to the charity, Pharmacist Support, and I am pleased to help in any way I can.

This book demonstrates the power of social media in bringing people together from around the World. This book shows just how small the world really is.

Preface

I started blogging in August 2011. It started off serious but then rapidly descended into mirth. I was encouraged to blog by @DrugMagister who is a pharmacist on twitter. I am anonymous because I thought it would allow me to say things that I can't as me.

I had the idea to write the book in June 2012. A similar book had been published earlier in the year. A pharmacist put an advert in the Journal four years ago asking for anecdotes and it took him four years to get published.

I decided to attempt one too and add in some of my blogs. People have been so helpful and I will never be able to fully repay them. Chemist and Druggist magazine, Pharmacy magazine and P3 magazine let me appeal for anecdotes. I also used my blog, Twitter, LinkedIn and Facebook too. I was able to get some anecdotes from the 'Pharmacy Forum' and 'Locum Voice' websites. Twitter helped me choose the title. Many thanks to Helen Root for coming up with it.

Pharmacy is currently in the middle of a Great Depression. I believe the profession needs cheering up and this book is my attempt to do that. It also has a reputation of being boring by non-pharmacy people and probably by a few people in the business too.

Our job is serious and professional. We care about our patients. We also have a sense of humour and the ability to laugh at ourselves, which I believe is important. Other professions in the UK have produced funny books but not ours yet. The exception is the book by @DrugMonkey but that is American.

The book is primarily aimed at people who work in pharmacy. However, I believe that that other healthcare professionals and indeed the general public will enjoy the book and perhaps learn a little bit more about our role. I have included a glossary which briefly explains any pharmacy specific terms. More detailed explanations can be found via Google.

So, here we are in January 2013 and the book is complete. Thanks to Lucy Pitt for the great front cover and all her help. Also thanks to Jonathan Mason for the foreword. I hope this is not the end of Mr Dispenser as I have more stories to tell. I will do so as long as people want me to. The book is intended to make people laugh and is not intended to offend anyone. 5% of sales are going to the Pharmacist Support Charity. Thank you for reading!

Mr Dispenser

Twitter

The following chapters are made up of tweets from several people or in the case of the last one involve several people from twitter. If it was not for twitter, I would not have started blogging and this book would never have been written.

I love twitter. Where else could you eavesdrop on a stranger's conversation, join in, argue with them, insult them and leave without a punch?

Twitter is a social networking tool. The messages that are posted are called tweets. Tweets are a maximum of 140 characters long. There are some very funny pharmacy people on twitter. The short nature of the message forces people to be direct, straight to the point and often very funny. Their names are preceded by a @ symbol.

Pills Part 1: I Don't Understand

Drugs have unusual names and can be hard to pronounce. Every day, working in a community pharmacy, we hear such wild and wacky pronunciations for a wide range of drugs – and they never cease to bring a smile to our faces. Patients are normally the main culprit of these major oral malfunctions, although it is not unheard of for pharmacy staff and even pharmacists to get it wrong from time to time too. As an example, someone asked me for some coleslaw cream today, and then I heard a fellow colleague ask for diasepan.

The Electronic Medicines Compendium has produced a medicine guides for patients. These also include the correct way to pronounce the drug. http://www.medicines.org.uk/guides "But how many patients have this at home to peruse, so we can't really blame them can we!?"

For example, Bendroh-flu-meth-eye-ahzide

Co-codamol

@Jonesy147: My grandmother used to say 'co-dominal' rather than co-codamol.

@Clareylang: Codramol.

Bendroflumethiazide

@SowTomorrow: Try keeping a straight face at an old lady who says "it's those tablets that sound like 'Bend Me Over The Fireside'!"

@impure3: I think bendro-whatsit is the most common.

Clopidogrel

@arleniebeanie: ClopiDOGrel!

@jonathanmason: Cloppy dog rell

@mrdispenser: Sloppydogrel.

Paracetamol

@alkemist1912: I'm sure one of my older patients asks for - Barry-shit-em-alls.

@kevfrost: Honourable mention for paracetamoxybendrofruseneomyocin?

Ibuprofen

@SusieMinney: Ibooprofen (from a fellow pharmacy technician).

@HelenRoot: Izobuzafen.

@pillmanuk: Eye-boo-pho-fen.

Omeprazole

@Clareylang: Ompazol.

Louise Isobel Henry: Omiprazolly.

@googlybear84: Diposlack Ointment (Diprosalic), Primigone (Piriton) & Calvaline Cream (Calamine).

@PatelSuk: Naftidoodidaties (naftidrofuryl).

@jonathanmason: I had a patient who referred to her "niffy dip ins" (Nifedipine). My old gran referred to Movelat as move-it gel.

@helenRoot: And the obvious anus-ol.

@tonyrob77: Also like Cacit pronounced as 'Kackit' and Fybogel pronounced as 'Fi-boh-gull'.

@darkvignette: I once got asked for some Robin Cousins cough medicine (Robitussin).

@tonyrob77: I always remember an old lady asking me for 'Methadone Tonic' (she meant Metatone of course).

@SowTomorrow: Ferocious sulphate.

@Suepharm: I had an elderly gent asking for Neck. It finally turned out to be Head and Shoulders.

@EmilyJaneBond82: CandyStatton (Candesartan).

@Lauraberrycakes: Lansarope (as in sounds like the place Lansarote) for Lansoprazole!

@frandavi99: I-prat-opium.

@cathrynjbrown: Hali-bori-orange as well.

@mraparmar: I've got a patient who's adamant her blood pressure meds are called "Rap-ri-mil"…I don't have the heart to tell her she's wrong.

@arleniebeanie: I have also had dippymole instead of Dipyridamole once!

@mumgonecrazy: Flufloxacillin.

@Planet_Jackie: One guy asked for his 'sillyarse' tablets……he meant Cialis.

@MaryP58: Slimvastatin – so close. The marketing team missed a trick there.

@pillmanuk: A-rato-va-stan.

@alkemist1912: Lactu-loose!!!

@Selinahuihoong: Celebrate instead of Celebrex.

@Cathrynjbrown: I always enjoy monkeylast.

@Planet_Jackie: An old lady handed me a note, she'd written down her medication to be repeated. It said 'Lovethyroxine'.

@Clareylang: Parrot (Pariet).

Wendy Finney: Carbellomarzipan [Carbamazepine]!

Rebecca Ross: My dispenser called Pregabalin 'preg balling'.

@TheCynicalRPh: My day shift pharmacist says we have a patient with cocksucky virus. He meant Coxsackievirus.

Sue L: I had a request for Sod You cream---turned out to be Sudocrem.

@Pharm_Thoughts: Sim-a-va-satin instead of sim-va-statin. Meto-pro-lawl instead of me-toe-pra-lawl (even pharmacists say this one incorrectly!).

Neelm: My dispenser calls lamotrigine = lamborghini, tibilone = Toblerone. "Am-I-triptyline?". " I don't know, are you?!"

Mr T: An old lady rang up to order her Rx on Monday and asked for opium strips (Optium Plus).

@mraparmar: Had a patient come in earlier asking for her "Lans-appraisal" [Lansoprazole].

@Zams123: Funniest thing I've ever heard from a customer: 'can I have some arse cream'?

Grumpy Old Woman: Last week someone wanted to buy 'kinky' tablets? "What are they for?" I asked, rather reservedly. Patient had no idea (!) but they'd been recommended by a friend and she'd bought it here before. She lived close by & went home to collect the old pack to show us. "This is it - kinky billobar" she said. She meant Ginkgo Biloba!

Zoggite: Then you've always got your Naffy-drawfuls (generic Praxilene.), and your simvastation for cholesterol... (has to be pronounced in a northern accent for the full effect!)

Grumpy Old Woman: I'm always fascinated by the variations on 'bendroflumethiazide'. It always starts with 'ben' & ends with 'ide', but the bit in the middle is usually a 'Tommy Cooper-esque' mumble of zzzz's!! (And they always say it with a straight face, with that utter confidence that everyone pronounces the word in exactly that same way!)

Zoggite: Upon collecting her Omeprazole script today, a lady told me that her GP reckoned she had "that helicopter-thing" (quote), and that's what was causing her stomach complaints.

Grumpy Old Woman: Baloney stockings (below knee), "I'm on Tiffin for blood pressure" (Tenif), "I take Allegro at night - you know, like the car" (Allegron)*, Fibre jelly (Fybogel) and little shitters (senna)!

Otterpond: My personal favourites are: "Aquarius cream" and "Aquacious cream" for aqueous cream, "Galveston" for Gaviscon, "Anus-hole cream" for Anusol, "Co-Co-Odomor tablets".

Zoggite: Talking of candesartan, I had a patient who insisted on pronouncing Amias in such a way that it sounded like "Eh my arse"... And the man who came in asking for some kotex [Otex]eardrops, and wondered why all the ladies in the shop were smiling! I've also had scripts for Anadin [Inadine] dressings, 9.5cm x 9.5cm, and Mephilix [Mepilex] tape 5cm.

Krystal: A very old one that I remember from my pre-reg days at a psychiatric hospital was one man who used to call his Orphenadrine tablets (Brand name Disipal) his 'dizzy pills'.

@pokey_pineapple: I had a guy asking for something for his chest constipation [congestion].

@impure3: "Amlobedean is for blood pressure yes?"

Indisangar: Just like the time when I was asked for Anus oil [Anusol], or even the time I was asked for discotears [Viscotears].

Sana: "Lemon chips" i.e. Lemsip.

MadcatLynn: Silly Ass [Cialis]and Happy trip-e-line [amitriptyline].

Pills Part 2: The effect of medicines on the olfactory system

Introduction

Olfaction is the sense of smell. A pharmaceutical drug, also referred to as medicine, medication or medicament, can be loosely defined as any chemical substance intended for use in the medical diagnosis, cure, treatment, or prevention of disease.

Aim

The aim is to find smelly drugs.

Method

A closed leading question was sent as a tweet to 370 people that follow @MrDispenser, asking to tell me about drugs that smell good or bad. No financial inducement was given due to Category M clawbacks. Ethics approval was refused. An application for funding was made and denied by the National Lottery. Consent was obtained via direct message for tweets to appear in this report.

Results

30 people replied. There were 7 males and 21 females. There were two people that I was unable to work out as the name was ambiguous and their profile picture was not a face picture.

My tweet was retweeted once. Two people did not give consent for their tweets to appear. Two did not reply so consent was given on their behalf.

Original tweet and replies

@mrdispenser: My staff members tell me that Depakote smells like cannabis.

@zams123: Depakote does smell like cannabis.

@L1ttlepetal: My dispenser ex bar manager said it smells like stale beer.

Neo-Mercazole

This was very popular and my personal favourite too!

@josephbush: Cannot beat Neo-Mercazole.

@indisangar: Smells like strawberry milkshake.

@susieminney: Carbimazole smells of milkshake.

Celevac

Another popular choice.

@laura_anne182: Prefer Celevac. I am a serial tub-sniffer.

@JustHelenYeah: Celevac has to be the best for smell and colour.

@Mushypea: Celevac is just like strawberry milkshake.

Bendroflumethiazide 2.5mg

This is the Ronseal of tablets.

@laura_anne182: Bendroflumethiazide 2.5mg (tubs of 500) smells like a chair in an old folk's home.

@indisangar: Bendroflumethiazide smells like urine, kind of appropriate, isn't it?

@jommcmillan: Bendroflumethiazide smells like what they do.

@cathrynjbrown: Bendroflumethiazide is bad.

@susieminney: Bendroflumethiazide smells like stale urine. It's ironic really.

@zams123: I like the musky smell of bendroflumethiazides!

Relifex

This was also popular.

@catrionabrodie: Nabumetone (especially Relifex) smells like butterscotch.

@alkemist1912: Relifex smell of butterscotch.

@Mushypea: Relifex was like butterscotch.

@cathrynjbrown: Relifex is good.

Vitamin B

This was a controversial tablet.

@PatelSuk: Can't believe no one's mentioned Vitamin B compound. It's weirdly addictive.

@Anj17: I don't like vitamin B. It smells.

@susieminney: I love the smell of vitamin B in any shape or form.

Vitamin caps BPC

Another controversial one.

@laura_anne182: Funny how the smells can grow on you. I am now quite fond of the stinky vitamin caps.

@lilygidley: Vitamin caps are like Bovril.

@JoMyatt: I love vitamin caps BPC.

@zams123: Vitamin BPC caps smell horrible.

@josephbush: Vitamin caps are Bovrily goodness.

@NeelmSaina: Vitamin BPC capsules have a Marmite smell.

@cathrynjbrown: Vitamin caps BPC are bad.

Antibiotics

Strong views on these common drugs.

@Anj17: The banana amoxicillin is yummy.

@NeelmSaina: Cephalexin capsules are bad.

@Sairah_Banu: Flucloxacillin smells like 1p sherberts.

@Mushypea: Flucloxacillin caps smell like sulphur.

@cathrynjbrown: Flucloxacillin capsules are bad.

@laura_anne182: Ciproxin suspension smells like Barratts Fruit Salads.

@adamplum: Love the smell of flucloxacillin mixture.

@clareylang: The flucloxacillin liquid is completely the opposite of the capsules.

@cathrynbrown: Oh yes, the waft of Amoxil or Distaclor powder as you pour the water in.

@clareylang: Augmentin Duo smells well nice.

@susieminney: Cephalosporins smell of cat urine.

@becky_ross_23: Co-danthramer suspension smells exactly like tinned peaches.

Aspirin

The smell is explained with science!

@zams123: Aspirin 75mg dispersible smells of salt and vinegar crisps.

@clareylang: Aspirin really does smell like that.

@adamplum: Because acetyl-salicylic acid breaks down to acetic acid.

Miscellaneous

@pillmanuk: Spironolactone used to smell of minty urine.

@xrayser: Ferrous Sulphate smells of Christmas pudding with Brandy Butter

@tinaallsup: Neoral smells very strongly of beer. No complaints.

@pakili1981: Lamotrigine smells like lollies.

@Sareenuh: Vicks VapoRub smells great.

@mgcmitchell: Calpol yum yum.

@mgcmitchell: Pabrinex, TPN, and coal tar are bad.

@Sairah_Banu: Fentanyl patches smell really weird.

@jommcmillan: Anybody remember Junifen? Used to smell like lemon puff biscuits.

@pillmanuk: NEVER smell Heminevrin liquid.

@misspill: Never break a full bottle in the dispensary either.

Two people have said that Mecysteine smells horrible like rotten eggs!

27 drugs were mentioned.

Discussion

Drugs smell. Vitamin caps BPC was the most commented drug. Relifex and Celevac were the best smelling drugs. Bendroflumethiazide was the worst smelling drug.

Future research

Facebook should be used as a research tool too.

Conclusion

Medicine Use Reviews [MURs] will never be boring again.

References

Wikipedia.

Comment

@weeneldo: Co-codamol 30/500 smells like a McChicken sandwich. Also, here's a true fact, manufacturers employ someone specifically to fart into tubs of flucloxacillin and cefalexin. Depakote doesn't just smell like weed, it smells like the sweat of someone who smokes a lot of weed. I believe the smell of Vit B12 is best described as "Umami" (look it up if you don't know what I'm talking about; knowledge is power. Although try telling that to British Gas). If you've ever smelled a Zoton Fastab, you'll know they're wonderful. Jilly Goolden has nothing on me. (apart from those Polaroids, but as long as I get the money to the park by 7pm it'll be OK).

Thrills

You wouldn't think that there were many thrills in pharmacy....

Thrill of a cuppa

Finding the time in a busy day to drink a hot cup of tea is impossible.

Thrill of Orlistat (weight loss drug)

A long term 'manufacturer can't supply' drug coming back into stock makes fat people jollier.

Thrill of being cheeky

Buying cakes for staff that are on a diet and putting sugar in someone's Diet Coke can.

Thrill of obscure university legend

@onepintwong: I was told at university that we would very rarely see vet scripts. Today, we got a vet script for 2100 850mg metformin tabs. I kid you not.

@Unicorn__FTW: I served a captain of a vessel last week. Another thing we were told at university that would practically never happen.

Thrill of the NHS

The best thing about the NHS is using my ETP smart card to get NHS discount at Nandos!

Thrill of lying to management

Darshana Thaker: Playing hide and seek with a regional manager because the store manager hasn't told him she's booked me.

Thrill of reading mucky books

I did four Emergency Hormonal Contraception (morning after pill) consultations in one day. Too much reading of a certain book was the cause.

Thrill of perfect dispensing

You get a prescription for amoxicillin 250mg x 15 capsules. You go to the shelf and there is a split box with exactly 15 capsules in and a leaflet too!

Thrill of asking out a dispenser

Abs: So one of my dispensers came out of the consultation room after supervising an addict with a look of shock on her face! The addict had suggested they go out on a date. He had written her the sweetest love note. I had to have a word with the addict the next day fortunately he was very understanding and apologetic. He does seem to have turned life around though and has a girlfriend now.

Thrill of denying people alcohol on Christmas day

@Babir1981: Do I feel bad about telling people that they can't drink alcohol with metronidazole today (Christmas Day)? Nope.

Thrill of catching a shoplifter

@dropboy: Does watching a program on shoplifting count as Continuing Professional Development? I need to catch them before closing time. I feel like Magnum PI.

Thrill of saying it to staff (in my head)

If you don't behave, I will stick my foot so far up your ass; my athlete's foot will give you oral thrush. I also call some of my staff Team Menopause, when they can't hear me.

Thrill of talking about patients

I like to play, 'Guess which patient looks like they could be a serial killer?'. I haven't got one right yet though thankfully.

@PrettyGirlRock: Sometimes we play patient snog, marry, and avoid.

@googlybear: I like to play "which patient actually has a genuine right to claim free prescriptions?", touchy subject though.

Thrill of sarcasm

I find it really hard not to be sarcastic sometimes. I have to hold my tongue. Like when patients ask where they need to sign on the back of a script. I can't help pointing and saying 'just where it says sign here!'

Thrill of war wounds

I once had two men comparing their triple heart bypass scars in the pharmacy.

Thrill of a dishy doc

@sarayummymummy: Ok, we have a very yummy Dr at our practice that I call Mr Darcy as he reminds me of him from Bridget Jones Diary! He already knows I have a soft spot for him ;-) & we have a good laugh about it! Anyways the girls in the pharmacy decided to tell him that I call him Mr Darcy in the pharmacy. One day I was in the back of the dispensary & I turn around and there he is standing there in his white Mr Darcy shirt with a big GRIN! He tells me: " Sara I thought I was more a George Clooney than a Mr Darcy?" my reply was "No Dr, Mr Darcy rocks in my books!" We had a good giggle and a laugh and let me tell you all since then everyone including his practice staff calls him Mr Darcy when I'm around including me! It certainly puts a nice spin on things.

Thrill of not getting a punch by patients

@weslangley: Ever tried the name game? Try calling a patient's name out in the funniest voice you think you can get away with. Also someone dares you to work a phrase or word into the next conversation. My favourite 'word the phrase into the consultation' is "my cats called Elvis"

@alkemist1912: Cheap thrills - mispronouncing patients' names badly. Making awkward customers wait for ages and ages and ages and when they moan tell them you called their name out 20 minutes ago. Making people who talk loudly and constantly on their phones wait until THEY finish their pointless calls.

Thrill of a bonus at work

@catrionabrodie: One place I worked in paid a masseuse to come in every 6 months to help us all.

@weeneldo: How can you forget "Thrill of a Good Sit Down" or "Thrill of Finally Getting to Go to the Toilet"? Best thrill though? When you get a 6 page prescription handed in and your heart sinks...before realising 5 pages are just repeat reorder forms! You kind of feel like you've actually achieved a minor victory.

Pharmacy Spills

People who work in pharmacy are pretty clumsy. What have you spilled in the pharmacy?

Methadone

@frandavi99: I discovered Methadone original makes your shirt go stiff as cardboard when it dries! I spent the day being described as a drug addict's lollipop.

@MrDispenser: I had a 500g tub of Diprobase cream fall from a shelf, miss my head and smash a conical with 100ml methadone. I had just qualified. I started laughing. Then I started crying.

@frandavi99: Smashing a conical is a big sin!

@catrionabrodie: I watched an AAH driver break some methadone once and the staff made HIM clear it up.

@Allucha: Methadone spills are horrid. I had 60ml spill all over myself one morning due to a poorly closed bottle. It stunk all day.

@Saij_J: Staff member spilled methadone all over counter. Locum spent whole morning trying to figure out how much was lost.

@Andychristo: Don't forget the delivery driver who dropped and smashed 12 methadone bottles.

Lactulose

@catrionabrodie: I think the worst thing to spill is Lactulose, absolute nightmare to clean...

@impure3: A full 500ml of methadone on a tiled floor and a glass bottle of lactulose on a carpeted floor. Guess which one was easier to clean? Yep! We had to have someone replace the carpet tiles for the other mess! I had been employed about a week. Oops!

@StandByPharmacy: Lactulose - a tiled floor remains sticky for months, no matter how well it is cleaned.

@The_Buffy_Bot: Lactulose. Bloody awful stuff!

Five-second-rule twitter conversation

@MrDispenser: I have spilled a bottle of tablets as I tried to put the lid on in view of the patient which was awkward. She did not believe in the five second rule.

@frandavi99: Two second rule can't be applied there sadly.

@Clareylang: We have the three second rule.

@impure3: We say three.

@MrDispenser: Is it the 2, 3 or 5 second rule?

@clareylang: Well we have 3 but guess it depends how strongly you feel about spills of pills lol!!! But really it's the 0 second rule!

@frandavi99: Depends how long it takes you to rescue it!

@Pillmanuk: Depends on the value of the spilt tablets. Some can have a five minute rule when they are over £100. Of course not, I was being silly. Everyone knows that the rules doesn't apply to them

Gaviscon

@Lauraberrycakes: Spilt Gaviscon isn't fun!

@gemcymru: Aniseed Gaviscon ...gloopy!

@Gemmieangel: A 500ml bottle of Gaviscon as my Area Manager walked in and the pharmacy had a carpet.

Coffee twitter conversation

@pill_saurus: Once I spilled a whole cup of hot coffee and almost 3-4 shelves of medicines were colourfully decorated!

@frandavi99: You wasted coffee!?

@pill_saurus: Yes, sacrilege and was so embarrassed as it was just my first week in the Pharmacy

@frandavi99: Was it just a very badly made coffee?

@pill_saurus: Didn't even get to the point of tasting it. Just picked the cup and was trying to grab a corner and spilled.

Cod Liver Oil

@frandavi99: I had a dispenser that knocked a bottle of cod liver oil over, smelt so bad we sent her home!

@Sianibarny: A 500ml bottle of cod liver oil! On a very hot day. No air con! I imagine the pharmacy still smells fishy 10 years on!!

Antibiotic Suspension

@Lauraberrycakes: We had a locum shake a bottle of reconstituted amoxicillin all over a computer keyboard and herself. It was at the start of the day, she had a cream top on so had bright yellow marks all day & new keyboard was needed!

@HelenRoot: I hate spilling antibiotics It usually gets under the keyboard and amongst your prescriptions.

@alkemist1912: A pre-reg once started shaking erythromycin syrup with the lid not fully on!!!!!!!!! What a mess!!

@JV_Roberts: Cefalexin, made it up (just add water) changed lid for a Click Lock then shook=pink spots all over my white shirt!

Tablets

@Wojciethromycin: I tend to always spill furosemide 20's...the smallest tablets we have in our pharmacy of course.

@HelenRoot: 1000 pot of ferrous gluconate on the floor! Like an episode of Total Wipeout.

@Uzzi_RM: A yet-to-be-sealed blister pack filled with various drugs.

Non-pharmacy

@weslangley: The beans!

@Kevfrost: Blood.

@alkemist1912: Various people over the years spilled their guts in the pharmacy sink!!!!!!!! YUK

@MilnerMichael: Blood when opening amps for destruction!!

@Sybil_Ramkin: Blood, sweat and tears!

Miscellaneous

@frandavi99: Not me but a locum dropped some amlodipine suspension (special) worth £300.

@allucha: Water from a (thoroughly rinsed) methadone bottle that was being used as a vase for flowers from one of our temperamental patients. The funny thing is that the flowers lasted well over three weeks! Two bunches; we put one in a normal bottle, and one in sugar free.

@impure3: Oh, a big tub of aqueous cream on a blue carpet. Messy!

@Cocksparra: A well packed bag. Smashed a bottle of Medinol, in slow motion for some reason and sounded like someone got shot.

@07sat: Lactulose, paracetamol suspension, bisacodyl tabs and pesky vitamin caps - thankfully not all in the same day!

@Darkvignette: Remember seeing a fellow student at university shake a 2 litre Winchester of Calpol with no lid. Very messy and quite pink!

@Miss___DJ: Colpermin capsules, then stood on a few, whole place smelt of peppermint!

@Pillpusheruk: Methadone, Gaviscon and lactulose.

@JV_Roberts: Just spilled Magnesium Hydroxide today, horrible stuff instantly clumps in measuring vessel, then plop! All over the counter!

@ShabnamMirza: One thing is for sure, Night Nurse liquid is still bright green when it hits the floor.

@HelenRoot: TCP on a carpeted shop floor. I once dropped three kids' bubble baths on a floor. There was foam everywhere as we tried to clean.

@catrionabrodie: One Saturday, my Counter Assistant spilt a shower gel and shampoo all over the floor and proceeded to mop.

Dubious Pharmacy Facts

1] @MrDispenser: Paracetamol is stronger than aspirin because it's a higher strength.

2] @MrDispenser: Calpol turns your wee into a pink suspension.

3] @MrDispenser: All drugs cost 5p. The remaining £7.60 goes into the pharmacy cake fund.

4] @MrDispenser: Boots also sell shoes.

5] @David_Loughlin: There's no one else in the shop so you're doing nothing else behind there.

6] @MrDispenser: That medicine is not out of stock. It's just on the top shelf and I'm too tired to stretch.

7] @MrDispenser: Every consultation room has a Jacuzzi.

8] @David_Loughlin: That brand doesn't work as well as the expensive one.

9] @MrDispenser: We only tell the receptionist that it's urgent and we need to speak to the GP. We actually want to discuss Corrie.

10] @MrDispenser: The only legal requirement on a CD script is a cool signature.

11] @rmoomin1: The male member of staff is always the pharmacist.

12] @louis_Purchase: You can really sell me that hydrocortisone cream to use on my face.

13] @MrDispenser: If you do an MUR, the MUR queen puts 50p under your pillow.

14] @MrDispenser: The three day co-codamol usage limit is just the best before date.

15] @rmoomin1: Preparation H is totally licensed for wrinkles.

16] @cathrynjbrown: And for after tattoos.

17] @kevfrost: All pharmacies are required to have a mortar and pestle. The counter assistants use it to prepare lunch.

18] @M4lh1: Uncollected Fortisip and gluten free foods go towards the Christmas buffet.

19] @MrDispenser: Pharmacists will sell Piriton for use in dogs.

20] @MrDispenser: Pharmacists don't need to know your full medication history. They are just being nosy.

21] @Jonesy147: Methadone is just green Calpol. It's all about the placebo effect.

22] @Louis_Purchase: I take my medication differently to the prescribed instructions because the Doctor told me to.

23] @cleverestcookie: Of course this medicine's effective, it's priced at £30.

24] @The_Buffy_Bot: Oh the doctor prescribed it? It must be right then, pay no attention to me.

25] @Jonesy147: The CD register only exists because pharmacists are so forgetful.

26] @m4lh1: My GP knows I take codeine & Nytol every day, just sell it me.

27] @cleverestcookie: Threw away your tramadol by mistake? Of course I can let you have 300. No charge either!

28] @MrDispenser: The addict really had 4 granddads that passed away.

29] @The_Buffy_Bot: Yes you're right; the branded version IS more effective.

30] @shazinw: When the lights are off in the pharmacy, this means we are playing hide & seek in the dark, not that the pharmacy is closed.

31] @googlybear84: Having a Viagra stuck in your throat will actually give you a stiff neck for hours.

32] @Jonesy147: "Homeopathy definitely works; I read it in the Daily Mail."

33] @The_Buffy_Bot: The CD register only exists because pharmacists can't be trusted not to help themselves.

34] @fuzzdammit: The pharmacy down the road gave me amoxicillin without prescription.

35] @m4lh1: Boyfriend: Girlfriends busy, I'll just pick up Levonelle for her. She's used it before, it'll be fine.

36] @MrDispenser: Pharmacists don't make fun of patients on twitter.

37] @MrDispenser: You can submit tweets as CPD.

38] @googlybear84: Shop staff members know nothing about the products they sell, and only recommend the ones they've actually used personally.

39] @rmoomin1: I take you more seriously when you name drop your second cousin twice removed who's a nurse and knows best.

40] @kevfrost: 5mL of amoxicillin, clarithromycin, ciprofloxacin, trimethoprim and metronidazole suspensions count for 5-a-day-fruits.

41] @sam4715: We only offer a managed repeat scheme to make more money. We tick everything on the repeat without asking the patient.

42] @danthedealer: Only the pharmacist is able to reorder your prescription over the telephone.

43] @MrDispenser: GPhC will never follow you on Twitter.

44] @MrDispenser: The white repeat slip is a legal prescription.

45] @hedferguson: Yes it will only take me 5 minutes to do your 20 item script but we're busy playing monopoly out the back.

46] @Cleverestcookie: All pharmacists chose pharmacy because they weren't clever enough to do medicine.

47] @MrDispenser: Pharmacists don't need to eat lunch and this prevents them from needing a shit and keeps waiting times down.

48] @Salsira: MURs take 5 minutes, doesn't matter if you are on two medicines or ten.

49] @lauraberrycakes: Of course I can stand and chat about (insert non-relevant topic) when there is a queue of people waiting.

50] @googlybear84: "Yes, I'm writing it down right now to order for you" whilst answering elusive Times crossword clue!

Tips for New Pharmacists

@JonF: Don't believe anything an addict tells you.

@mrdispenser: Don't sell two Ventolin Evohalers for £7

@mrdispenser: Pharmacy is a small world. I probably went to university with someone that you know.

@cathrynjbrown: Mobile phones are a handy tool, but make sure you're not just texting/tweeting your mates.

@thorrungovind: It's mandatory to wear a full lab coat, surgical mask and safety glasses whenever you are in the pharmacy.

@thorrungovind: Thou shall not call drugs 'sweets'.

@thorrungovind: Thou shall not steal pens from drug reps.

@thorrungovind: You must be able to recite the BNF backwards.

@josephbush: Never believe any health story that appears in the Daily Mail. Correction, never believe anything in the Daily Mail.

@laura_anne182: When doing locum/relief work, don't bother bringing an expensive fancy pen. You will never see it again.

@thorrungovind : A customer WILL come in and ask you to draw the chemical structure of Aspirin.

@l_Q_Balls: Start watching X Factor, Big Brother & any other garbage on television if you want to join in the conversations on Monday morning.

@rmoomim1: If there's a lull in customers on a busy day, go to the loo, even if you only need to go a little bit.

@mrdispenser: All staff like fresh cream cakes, especially those on diets.

@david_loughlin: Don't be afraid to say no. And don't be afraid of the kettle!

@NavinSewak: If a doctor says 'trust me I'm a doctor' be very suspicious!

@weeneldo

-Learn to love newsagent sandwiches; you'll be eating a lot of them.

- Get a job with a large multiple or supermarket. Growing up you had 16 years of being spoken to like a child, so you've got great experience of their management style already!

- Calpol cures everything.

- Read the directions on labels. Imagine the instructions are a law. Could Johnny Cochrane get someone off with breaking that law? If so, it's too ambiguous. Rephrase and repeat process.

- You can't access patients' medical records. Receptionists can. You can't speak to the GP. Receptionists can. You can't sleep at night. Receptionists can.

- Assume all dental prescriptions are incorrect until proven otherwise. Also applies to controlled drug prescriptions.

- Five minutes is a crazy amount of time to wait for six prescription items. Patients will usually roll their eyes and say they'll come back if asked to wait this long.

- Don't bother advising patients receiving metronidazole to avoid alcohol. None of them ever drink anyway.

Remember: if a prescription asks for 15 Gaviscon Infant Sachets, dispense a box of 30 doses. This is because the box saying 30 doses actually means 15 dual dose sachets as each sachet is actually 2 sachets and therefore a quantity of 30 on the box is equivalent to 15 on the script. Also, despite the box saying 30 doses, it may only contain 15 doses depending on the weight and age of the patient. So a 30 dose box (written as 15 sachets on the script) might last 15 doses or it might last 30 doses. So to summarise: if the script says 15, dispense a 30 box containing 15 dual sachets which may be either 30 or 15 actual doses. You might think this seems complicated. It isn't, it's actually just really stupid.

I have a confession to make. I have a super power. Well every pharmacist has it as well. It's the power of super-hearing. I did not ask for it. Nor did I receive any training for it. I did not spend hours during my pre-registration year blindfolded to heighten my sense of hearing. It happened as soon as I qualified. I developed the ability to hear things without realising. As my Uncle Ben once told me; "With great power comes great responsibility."

I could be having a conversation in the dispensary and then all of a sudden, my spidey sense would start tingling and I would be able to hear that I needed to intervene and I would swing over the dispensary bench and come to the rescue at the counter. Men have the power to switch off this gift/curse. It's called selective hearing. I stop using it when the dispensary conversation turns to women's problems or (*insert whichever reality TV is on at the moment*).

Pharmacy Films

These are not in any order! This was started by @CandDChris. Special thanks to @pillmanuk for assisting in the compilation.

1] @CPPEGFlavell: Gone with the Windeze.

2] @EPSPharmacist: The Rx Files.

3] @RSDave: The 39 steps to re-accreditation.

4] @RSDave: Debbie does Diazepam.

5] @L1ttlepetal: A Clockwork Fybogel Orange

6] @RSDave: Senna.

7] @josephbush: Mission Impossible V: Procuring Orlistat.

8] @Xrayser: Bridge Over The River Kwai garlic.

9] @kevfrost: Se7en day scripts for Dosettes.

10] @impure3: The Fast and the Furosemide.

11] @lil_rea_rea: The Dark Nytol.

12] @MCPharmS: Goldeneye Drops.

13] @abitina: MUR on the orient express.

14] @mrdispenser: Die hard with a Viagra.

15] @jasonpeett: ACEi Ventura Pet detective.

16] @MCPharmS: Star Wars: Revenge of the Cyst.

17] @SowTomorrow: Fargocalciferol.

18] @aisha_adnan: Joan of Arcoxia.

19] @pill_O_saurus: The Good, The Bad and The Urgotul.

20] @ChaChaChandni: Harry Potter and the Chamber of Controlled Drugs.

21] @jasonpeett: Star Trek 3: The Search for Stock.

22] @jasonpeett: Independents Day.

23] @manolo_ko: 28 Days Later (Repeat Prescription.)

24] @RSDave: No Flomax for Old Men.

25] @tobyhiggins: Kill Pill.

26] @mumegonecrazy: Dirty Dispensing.

27] @mrdispenser: Ferrous Sulphates Day Off.

28] @tonyrob77: Catch Me If You Canesten.

29] @EmilyJaneBond82: Twin Peak Flow Meters.

30] @katie7h: Avatarginact.

31] @mrdispenser: Saving Ryan's Private Prescription.

32] @kevfrost: Dude, where's my Carbamazepine?

33] @KrishOza: How to lose a Rx in 10 days.

34] @EPSPharmacist: American History Rx.

35] @mrdispenser: Dial M for MUR.

36] @GwavaSalim: Get MURs or die tryin.

37] @amyotway: MUR Due Date.

38] @tonyrob77: Lord of the Ring Pessaries.

39] @PatelSuk: Live and Let Dyazide.

40] @NeelmSaini: Home Asilone.

41] @ChrisALangley: On the Trusses.

42] @CandDChris: The Great Escitalopram.

43] @amyotway: Lock, Stock and Two CD cabinets.

44] @tonyrob77: Wall-E45.

45] @tonyrob77: Escape to Victoza.

46] @EPSPharmacist: The Incredible Broken Bulk.

47] @googlybear84: Kick Aspirin.

48] @kevfrost: The Phenytoin Menace.

49] @JonnyB _at_RMP: Sister Actos.

50] @s9njay: Good Pill Hunting.

Waste Disposal

One of the things that I dread is when a patient appears with two bin bags full of returned medicines. However, I don't think they understand what they can and cannot return. The following have all been found in carrier bags full of patient returned medication:

@lauraberrycakes: False teeth.

@Mushypea: Underskirt.

@AdamPlum: Kaolin poultice.

@ilSuarez: Incontinence pants.

@kelbel69696969: Pharmacy bag stuffed with £15k.

@SusieMinney: Wrongly labelled/dispensing error of Concerta.

@wyldchild007: Old medication from 1972.

@Calorinee: Cat food.

@frandavi99: Keyring torch.

@darkvignette: A prosthetic breast, packaged in a gift box complete with ribbons.

@pharmorto: Stool sample.

@mumgonecrazy: Cigarettes and a small safe.

@bengalkitti: Old postcards, family photos, pairs of glasses, boxes of buttons and an old watch.

@Alansleith: A miniature malt whiskey.

For me, it's a full box of Tamiflu. It's good that a patient brings back unwanted medicines for us to safely dispose of but not so good when they hand in a prescription at same time for same thing!

Comments

Julie Goucher: Spooky! I processed a bag of medication for destruction about 3 years ago at a pharmacy in Devon. Inside was a box dispensed at a pharmacy that I had worked in, in Surrey during 1989. I glanced at the little dispensed and checked boxes and sure enough they were my initials! Happy memories!!

Sarah L: Nine years' worth of repeat slips, not a single one missing and all in order.

Cam: Somebody brought back about 50 (FIFTY) Cialis 20mg for destruction.

Nik: Bring in a big bag of old medicines, most still in their full original packs, dated from 1997 to be disposed of at the pharmacy. When asked if they contain any needles or controlled drugs respond "I don't know, the wife always looked after the dog's medication".

@googlybear: Hearing aids covered in wax, thick orange/brown wax!

Arlene Caldwell: Nothing strange but has to be empty medicine bottles amongst drug returns and drugs dating back to 1976!!

@weeneldo: I received a bottle of Gentian Violet from 1988 this year...a year older than me! I also once got a patient's scales for dealing weed in a bag of returns.

My Blogs

These are the blogs that do not involve people from twitter.

Why does it take so long to slap a label on a box?

1] Patient walks in and leaves the door open on a cold day.

2] Assistant puts down her 'Take-a-Break' magazine and looks up.

3] Patient hands assistant the prescription.

4] Assistant makes small talk and complains she has no money.

5] She asks if the patient pays or is exempt.

6] She takes a prescription charge off the patient.

7] Assistant tells patient all about her last holiday which was a cruise.

8] Assistant brings the prescription into the dispensary.

9] Prescription falls on the floor.

10] Dispenser can't pick it up due to her false nails.

11] Pharmacist picks it up.

12] Places it in a basket or onto a clip to indicate waiting.

13] Technician scans the barcode on the prescription.

14] ETP not working.

15] Labels it manually.

16] Checks if it's NCSO.

17] Broken bulk?

18] Eligible for New Medicines Service?

19] Due for MUR?

20] Proscript flags up that it is eligible for NMS.

21] Try to print out consent form.

22] No paper in printer.

23] Paper reloaded.

24] Labels generated.

25] Labels run out halfway through.

26] Labels are replaced.

27] Endorser not working.

28] Product dispensed.

29] Product handed to pharmacist along with the prescription.

30] Checks for signature.

31] In date?

32] Clinically appropriate?

33] Blacklisted?

34] Wrong formulation has been dispensed.

35] It is sent back for amending.

36] Re-dispensed.

37] Pharmacist loses his pen.

38] The whole pharmacy team looks for the pen.

39] Pen is found in pharmacist's trouser pocket.

40] Near miss log filled out.

41] Pharmacist hand endorses script.

42] Patient has a hard to pronounce name.

43] Pharmacist ponders whether the forename or surname is easiest to pronounce.

44] Pharmacist turns over script and sees that patient has paid for the prescription.

45] Shouts out patient's name.

46] Patient comes to counter.

47] Pharmacist tells patient that their 28 dispersible aspirin 75mg is cheaper to buy.

48] Patient is refunded and buys 100 x aspirin 75mg dispersible.

49] Pharmacist secretly upset at losing NMS

50] Patient leaves.

Some like it hot

Some people cannot function in the morning without some caffeine. The United Kingdom Tea Council (http://www.tea.co.uk/teafacts) states that 80% of office workers now claim they find out more about what's going on at work over a cup of tea than in any other way. The figure is 98% in pharmacy.

You go to some pharmacies and there is a hot drink offered to you as soon as you walk in; always a sign of a good pharmacy in my opinion. In others, you are pointed to the direction of the kettle and have to struggle to find a clean mug or a spoon that isn't brown. Sometimes it's so busy that no one makes a drink all day, (and probably no one speaks to you either) and you never go back to that pharmacy.

It may be wise to bring a travel mug with you as it's rare that you get to finish a full mug of the hot stuff. In fact a fully drunk mug of tea whilst still warm is seen as a sign of weakness in many pharmacies! My own philosophy is to drink hot blackcurrant or orange cordial. This is normally met with strange looks. Hot cordial is like a placebo Lemsip. Once it cools down though, you can still drink it. Cold coffee is vile.

Some people don't like making tea and always say that it's not their turn. Some pharmacies have a rota and SOP in place. This includes a list on the wall stating who has what. If you give Sarah black tea instead of white coffee, then the near miss log is helpfully on the wall too. People have their own mugs too. Some have their names or age on which is helpful.

A word of warning. I heard a story once of a locum who was very particular about his tea. The teabag first, then the hot water and then the milk. The order was important. One day he dared to question the dispenser about whether or not this regime had been followed. Needless to say, he was told in no uncertain terms what he could do if he wasn't happy with his tea and I can guarantee to this day thereafter, his tea was NEVER made following his formula.

If you time tea-making just right then a patient will always chime in that they want a cup of tea too. It is obligatory to laugh at this comment no matter how many times you have heard it. It's a rite of passage for the fourteen year old work experience boy to make tea for everyone. This is generally the first time they have ever made tea in their life and they need advising that you need to actually switch the kettle on to get a hot drink, remove the teabag before handing it to the Pharmacist, and use one or two sweeteners, not the whole tube .

Most pharmacies collect tea money from staff in order to finance hot beverages. One person is usually put in charge of this complicated and not to forget important task. Often Excel spread sheets are used to name and shame staff who conveniently forget to pay up.

Staff members in pharmacy are always on a diet so have no sugar and opt for three biscuits instead. On a good week of offers at the supermarket there may be sightings of hot chocolate and "fancy" caffeine options available at the Pharmacy. Upper class pharmacies offer soup. Bovril however, is not allowed in my pharmacy. Yuck!

The hot drink is one of the most enjoyable aspects of the day. Let's face it; coffee is like lubrication to the work flow, an essential uplift. In the future it may be possible to hook up freshly brewed coffee to the Methameasure machine. Staff would be allowed 200ml TDS after successful fingerprint recognition. I'm still waiting for the patent to be approved!

For a few brief seconds, when your lips touch the warmth of your mug and get soaked by the milkiness of your perfect cup of tea, you can forget about the chaos and imagine a better place.

Comparethepharmacy.com

Welcome to the new comparethepharmacy.com website.

The aim is to help patients choose which pharmacy to use based on key categories and choices.

All pharmacies in England, Scotland and Wales that agreed to join are on the website.

Please choose one of the options for each category.

a] Waiting times should be:

1] 20 minutes.

2] 10 minutes.

3] 5 minutes.

4] 1 minute [The pharmacy cannot guarantee the correct medicine though].

b] Pharmacist appearance:

1] Lab coat.

2] Suit.

3] Jeans.

4] Not bothered.

c] Deliveries:

1] Same day.

2] Next day.

3] Only during ad breaks of Jeremy Kyle.

4] Pharmacy does not deliver.

d] Staff conversation:

1] Miserable staff who don't speak.

2] Polite chit chat.

3] Interrogation from staff about your private life.

4] Gossip about other patients.

e] Prescription ordering method:

1] Phone.

2] In person.

3] Email.

4] Twitter.

5] Facebook.

f]MUR:

1] Happy to discuss medication with pharmacist.

2] Do not want to bother. I know what I'm doing.

3) I have one of those with the doctor; it's nothing to do with you.

g] NMS:

1] Happy to be contacted.

2] Stop bleeding ringing me!

3) I'll say yes just to get out, but then block your number.

h] I would like the consultation room to be used for:

1] Discussing my medication.

2] Showing the boil on my ass to the pharmacist.

i] The time that the pharmacist is allowed for lunch is:

1] No lunch.

2] Eat while standing up.

3] 20 mins.

4] 30 mins

j] I want my tablets to come in:

1] Capsules when the prescription states tablets.

2] The colour of my choice.

3] The manufacturer of my choice.

4] Chocolate flavour.

k] Patient satisfaction survey:

1] I am happy to fill it in.

2] I will tick random boxes.

3] Can't be bothered. The Pharmacy is crap. Would rather be in the pub.

l] Patient returns:

1] I will return all unused medication.

2] My next of kin will return all unused medication.

3) I would like a refund if I return my prescription medicines

m] Do you require a 24 hour Daily Mail article advice hotline?

1] Yes

2] No

Additional ideas from the world of Twitter

n] @NickThayer99:

The Pharmacy does / does not insist on prescriptions to dispense medication

o] @kevfrost:

For emergency supply they charge:

1] Cost + markup.

2) Rx charge.

c) Nothing, gullibly believing that a prescription will follow.

Your list of pharmacies will be emailed to you.

Thanks for using comparethepharmacy.com!

Gadgets in Pharmacy

[Inspired by Stephen Fry]

TV: Very few pharmacies have them. Good for promoting services and key messages. Also lets patients watch Jeremy Kyle whilst waiting for their prescription.

Laptop: Used for Methameasure and viewing restricted websites.

Landline: Best way to get stonewalled by a GP receptionist.

Pen: Losing one of these can increase waiting times.

Microwave: Essential for warming up last night's left overs.

Smartphone: Used for sneaky tweeting whilst the boss is not looking.

Digital camera: Passport photos.

Desktop computer: Can you imagine typing labels on a typewriter?

Electric Kettle: Most valuable gadget in pharmacy.

Fax: Used for receiving illegal CD prescriptions.

Retractable tape measure: Measuring for legs for hosiery

Stapler: Normally empty but invaluable.

Calculator: Used all the time after qualification.

Bathroom scales: Weighing customers before going on Lipotrim and for the weekly staff weigh-in.

Burglar Alarm: Keeps addicts out.

Vacuum Cleaner: Cleaning up mess left by naughty kids.

Answerphone: We have not got one but some customers insist that they left us a message on it.

Fan: Used for two days of the year when it's hot at work.

Shredder: Destroying confidential waste.

Scissors: This is used when dispensing split quantity of Stugeron.

Tablet counting machine: For those who can't operate a triangle.

McPharmacy

Pharmacy has a lot in common with fast food chains.

Here are five reasons:

1) Both have long waiting times. "Why is my burger/simvastatin taking so long?"

2) Generally you can't see the staff working in the kitchen/dispensary, but you can hear them talking.

3) Both (unfortunately) have drive-thru available.

4) Both run out of products and having no ice-cream/temazepam brings out different but strong emotions in people.

5) Both have 16-year old clueless Saturday assistants on the counter.

Exciting vacancy at Mr D's pharmacy

Mr Dispenser's pharmacy is a forward thinking organisation and is honoured to create a new position in pharmacy: **The Pharmacy Receptionist.**

-Must be a stubborn, miserable individual and have balls of steel (Not literally. See Dr.Christian if literally).

Skills

-Be able to take hours to answer incoming calls.

-Be able to handle being the first port of call for the patient.

-Ability to grill patients as to why they want to see the pharmacist.

-Telling patients that they won't be able to see the pharmacist until a week on Tuesday.

-Be assertive in deterring doctors wishing to speak to the pharmacist.

-Ability to provide pharmaceutical advice with no training provided.

-Be able to charge for sample bottles.

-Advanced communication skills to explain the pharmacist is busy, even when they can be seen drinking a cold cup of tea.

-Be able to refer patients to the GP as the pharmacist is busy.

-Be able to give out confidential information over the phone without checking who the caller is.

-Be able to look down on people.

-Salary: Minimum wage.

-Closing date: 1st April.

-Please apply via Twitter.

Can I take your order please?

On November 4th 2011, an article was published on the BBC NEWS website entitled, 'Receptionists 'key' to safe repeat prescription process'. This reported a study from the British Medical Journal.

Here are some quotes from it and my thoughts in bold:

'GP receptionists play a "hidden" role in ensuring patients get the correct treatments when they need them'

It's so hidden that no-one has ever seen it happen!

'Are receptionists the unsung heroes in general practice?'

No, it's the guy that collects the stool samples and takes them to hospital.

'Many were adept at using a formulary to match brand names with generic equivalents; they often telephoned patients to clarify ambiguous requests, and many kept (individual or shared) notebooks containing knowledge they had gleaned on the job'.

Maybe someone should invent a book that contains the names of drugs in it and bring it out twice a year? Or maybe they could send a similar one to surgeries every month!?!

'Some receptionists, the study found were aware of having to make up for the failings of their doctors'.

I suppose the four-year receptionist degree and having to pass a telephone exam to join the register and be regulated by the General Receptionist Society helps.

'Receptionists in some practices expressed concern that doctors did not check prescriptions thoroughly before signing'.

This could explain why a GP registrar prescribed 2L of paracetamol suspension to a baby.

'They believed that because of this they had a heavy responsibility to undertake safety checks themselves, although these were not recognised or remunerated'.

Safety checks?!? Is that checking blood results? Checking for interactions and contra-indications? GP receptionists get a basic wage but get a bonus payment for every time they stop a pharmacist from talking to a GP on the phone. Every surgery should employ a pharmacist to help with the repeat prescription process.

Staff Night Out

After a long week of dealing with awkward customers, the pharmacy team decided to go out for a meal on Saturday evening. We got there and were told that there would be a twenty minute wait. Understandably we got mad and vented our anger on the waitress.

We sat down and waited patiently. Ten minutes later, the senior technician shouted that we had been waiting twenty minutes. The waitress looked flustered and said that it was their busy period and they were short-staffed. That's not our problem!

There was another party waiting too. Once they heard our heckles, they joined in. We discussed how the service had gone downhill and how it was quicker in the restaurant down the road loudly so that the waitress could hear.

We were still waiting and a couple came in and got seated straight away. The senior counter assistant got up and complained! The couple had apparently been in before and were calling back. We did not believe a word and gave her a dirty look.

Finally, we got seated. The waitress came to take our order. I was busy talking on the phone and told her to come back for my order. Everybody else ordered.

Once my call was over, I had a look at the menu. I could not believe how expensive some of the items were. There is no way that I can afford this. I made this known to the waitress and then tweeted it on my new iPhone 5.

They did not have the food that I wanted in stock. They had ran out but would have some in tomorrow. I was not impressed at all. The junior tech stood glaring at the waitress all the time while we were waiting for our food. This speeds things up apparently.

Two of the waitresses were standing around talking about last night's television while we were waiting for our food. We could not see into the kitchen but could hear laughter. They were obviously not doing anything. How long does it take to slap a bit of food onto a plate?

The food was served. I asked for a word with the chef. He was busy. This annoyed me. The junior counter assistant was not happy with her tomato soup. She only likes Heinz brand. She told them that she would begrudgingly accept it this time but would take her business elsewhere if they did not keep her brand in.

The Chef finally came out. I asked for a word in private. I asked him how to get my Yorkshire puddings to rise. He did not seem impressed.

Oh well. Back to work on Monday to those awkward patients!

Waiting or Calling back

A comment from @L1ttlepetal on Twitter got me thinking about an extremely difficult question that we all ask patients numerous times an hour......."Are you waiting or calling back (CB)?"

You would think the only answers would be, 'waiting' or 'CB'. Maybe so in a perfect world, but no, that would be too easy. Sometimes it is a confusing yes, making me repeat the question.

Here is a community pharmacy definition of waiting: sit down, shut up and entertain yourself.

The term CB is most often ambiguous. Stepping out to the shop next door and coming straight back does not qualify as CB but it is the sign of an impatient waiter.

It seems in pharmacy that there are two extremes within the CB group. One being the few who nip out and come back impatiently assuming a quick exit can magically speed up the process of checking & dispensing.

RESULT: *rolling eyes*

The second group, return only to sit down quietly and they have already missed the calls of some pharmacists checking and shouting their name before placing the medicine away and half an hour later, the patient impatiently queries how long it's going to be. Half of this second group will wait and wait and dare not ask how long it's going to be until we ask them.

RESULT: *rolling eyes*

I must give an honourable mention to those who are waiting but wait in the car. For those with young kids, I am happy to bring the prescription out to them. For those who are parked illegally, their prescription seems to take longer for us to do. I have no idea why...

Some strange people ask not to wait but want it delivered. I try to persuade them to take ten minutes out of their daytime television, I mean busy schedule, and wait for it.

Others ask for deliveries but pop in for it instead. They ask where their medication is. We say, 'it's with the driver'. They ask, 'where is the driver?' We say that 'he's probably at your house love'.

Placing the CB or waiting script in the correct basket is the crucial step to avoid A SYSTEM COLLAPSE!!

Different pharmacies have their own systems, different coloured baskets, or hanging scripts in order, with further variations in filing for deliveries and MDS, this can be confusing for locums or even a technician with a hangover.

Other ways of reaching "A SYSTEM COLLAPSE" is placing the baskets in incorrect areas of the dispensary for the pharmacist to check.   The worst case scenario is filing a prescription away before dispensing, causing a prescription hunt upon the arrival of the patient.

RESULT: *panic at the pharmacy*

The final problem is when you haven't written down the time that the prescription was handed in. This results in queue jumpers and provides perfect opportunities for grumpy people to be...grumpy!

RESULT: *panic at the pharmacy*

This made me remember how at university, I once handed in my prescription to the local pharmacy and said that I would call back the next day. The girl on the counter seemed annoyed and asked, 'Why can't you wait?' The pharmacist looked at her in anger and asked 'Don't you think I'm busy enough???' and said to me that he would see me tomorrow.

Even if you are waiting or CB, it's never dull in pharmacy! I have some advice for patients. Don't taunt me by saying that you will be back for the prescription in five OR ten minutes as I will start making it up in four OR nine minutes depending on how I feel!

Naughty kids

This is not about Attention Deficit Hyperactivity Disorder. It is about the many naughty children that are brought into the pharmacies across the country by their parents and run wild.

A typical scenario is a 5-year old running around screaming and pulling boxes off shelves (not bottles if we are lucky). They are also infamous for treating lipsticks as glorified crayons, as they ruin the make-up section before jumping up and down on their seats with their muddy shoes. The brats don't like it when I wrestle the chlamydia/EHC/Erectile Dysfunction leaflets away from them whilst trying to be polite in front of their overly protective passive parents.

However some parents decide to solve this problem by keeping the child's hands occupied with doughnuts and sausage rolls whilst running around. I wonder to myself, are the kids like this at home? It's highly likely.

I am by no means advising spanking marathons in the pharmacy. That would create too much paperwork for me and is ethically wrong. I am merely asking for 'the look'.

'The look' was designed and patented by my mum when I was young. She deployed it whilst we were out and I misbehaved in public. 'The look' stopped me in my tracks. 'The look' meant that she was legally unable to strike me in public but if I carried on, she would have a 'discussion' with me at home. It always worked.

Also, parents, when naming your child, please bear in mind the pharmacy staff who will have to shout the name out one day. Keep it simple!!!! And then don't get annoyed when I mispronounce the name!

Some parents don't seem to care at all that their kids run riot in shops. Should we teach "the look"? ...my new pharmacy lifestyle advice for the mental stability of parents and pharmacists of little rascals.

Comments

Stephen Riley: Whilst working in a supermarket Pharmacy the store was hosting a party of local primary school children. They came over to the Pharmacy to say hello. One of the dispensers asked the children if they knew what colour a prescription was. To which one shouted,' I know they're blue!'

@weenoldo: Ask for a product for your child. When told it will cost £5.49, say "pfff, no way am I paying that!" They emerge from the shop next door two minutes later with 20 Benson and Hedges.

The Other Guys

Nurses, dentists and hospital doctors make GPs seem competent at prescribing.

Nurses

Many people think they are experts in dressings, sadly, they have been mistaken. It is extremely annoying to get a dressing prescription only to later find out they have written an incorrect size and doubly annoying when you have to send the prescription to NWOS. It is triply annoying when they don't answer their phone!

A nurse prescription for Dihydrocodeine 30mg tablets Four QDS naturally brought out the detective in me, feeling concerned I rang the nurse and it turned out that she had only prescribed the item because a patient had verbally told her a consultant had recommended that dose.

Back to the topic of dressings, nurses, yes nurses, are legally unable to prescribe a box of dressings, meaning any quantity more than three comes out of their back pockets. I also plead for patients not to believe a district nurse who says "I will order a prescription for you".

Dentists

These are professionals with a love for prescribing strange doses and out-of-bound drugs. I have seen Amoxicillin QDS [should be TDS], Amoxicillin tablets [don't exist!] and co-codamol on a dental script [Not allowed]. I have had many phone calls trying to explain the rules to them. Prescriptions regularly come through not stamped.

Dentists are also lazy. Take this for example; they write the dose but then get the receptionist to write the name and address on the prescription. The very lazy ones have stamps with the drug and dose on, so no handwriting involved, and no need for any extra pressure on those precious little tooth-extracting fingers.

A couple of months ago, a nice dentist prescribed two Temazepam 10mg tablets for an anxious patient prior to her dental procedure. He unfortunately increased her anxiety by forgetting to add 'For dental treatment only'! This is a legal requirement for 'CD' dental prescriptions.

Hospital doctors

These guys change the rules. They place the address labels over the part of the prescription that says that the outpatient prescription can only be dispensed in hospital. They refuse to print their name inside the very box that's asking for it. They also refuse to sign their name IN the signature box. This forces pharmacists to chase the hospital doctor through a maze of automated options and depressing music. The most items that I have seen on a handwritten hospital prescription is twelve.

A hospital prescription for Eurax Plus cream showed no results on my computer, Google, AAH, Alliance, NPA information department or from the company that produces Eurax. Once the secretary rang me back [Consultants never use the phone], she told me that the consultant had found Eurax Plus on the internet and decided to prescribe it....

@lifeonthepharm: Dentists can't get their heads around dates too. I've had today's date as a d.o.b and vice versa.

Andy Christo: Best Nurse prescription: Catheter: send one. When I phoned for the size, I was told to measure patient in shop!

Susie Minney: The dentist who prescribed Microgynon 30.

@Manj23: What about dentists always hogging the endorsement space?!!!

Locums Deserve Respect

Normally on a Saturday, I work in my own pharmacy. It gives me a chance to have a catch-up as it's generally quieter. This week, I was asked by the locum co-ordinator to work in a different branch. I had not worked at this branch for a couple of years, so I thought it would be nice to work there. Big mistake!!!

The morning started well and the two staff seemed pleasant. We did not do many items but it was all the problems in between that slowed everything down. Firstly, patients came back for items that were in that morning's AAH order. I looked through twelve AAH boxes to try to find a tub of Doublebase cream and then found it in the Alliance order!

Patient **A** brought in a prescription for Algesal cream and they were calling back. We did not have it in stock so I put it to one side for when Patient A came back.

Patient **B** came in for an owing from yesterday for Oestrogel. Unfortunately, it had not been ordered. Luckily, she was happy to wait until Monday.

The next prescription for Patient **C** made me chuckle: She wanted peppermint Glandosane but not peppermint Gaviscon and had stuck a Post-It note on the prescription. They liked peppermint but not for everything! A verbal instruction was not sufficient apparently.

Patient **D** collected a prescription but it was the wrong flavour of Paracetamol 6+ suspension. He does not like orange?!?! So I had to change all 1200ml. In the middle of this, Patient **E** rang to speak to the pharmacist and I said that I would ring them back. I only had 600ml so I gave an owing note. There was also another prescription for Gabapentin that should have been here. I looked on the computer and said that the last one was done a week ago. She said that she had only ordered it a few days ago and we should have collected it. She would ring the surgery on Monday morning.

The waiting time had increased to 10 minutes and one patient walked out in disgust?!?!

I rang Patient **E** back and there was no answer!

Patient **F** came in for an emergency supply of her dad's Dihydrocodeine tablets as he had forgotten to order them. I referred her to the emergency doctors who would be able to fax me a prescription.

Patient **E** rang back and had been prescribed some Zufal [Branded generic Alfusozin] tablets. We could not get hold of them and he was not happy. He was going on holiday on Wednesday. He kindly gave me the address of AAH Pharmaceuticals in Leeds for me to try on Monday [thanks!]. I explained that I would leave a note for the next pharmacist on Monday and that we would definitely ring him back on Monday. He would begrudgingly accept a different generic if we could not get Zufal [Script would need to be changed though].

Patient **A** came back. The prescription had disappeared?!?!? It was not where I had left it. We all searched everywhere for it. EVERYWHERE. It had vanished.

20 minute wait for prescriptions……

I had to profusely apologise and say that we would ring the surgery on Monday to get another prescription. As soon as we get a replacement [hopefully!] the bleeding thing will probably turn up!

Patient **F** came back for the Dihydrocodeine fax. It had not arrived yet….

Patient **G** rang up and said that he was waiting for his Clopidogrel. It was due to be delivered on Mondays. I said that I would bring it on my way home at 1pm. He was 94 years old so I felt generous!

Patient **H** said that there was no Ramipril tablets on her Mum's prescription from yesterday and wanted an emergency supply. I looked on the computer and which said that it had been labelled. I found out the prescription and it was on there. I asked her to confirm with her mum that she had definitely not had them. Not a lot I could do apart from re-dispensing it.

Patient **F** came back again. Still no fax. She rang the emergency doctors again. They had got our fax number wrong!

Patient **J** needed an emergency supply of Amlodipine....

The Dihydrocodeine fax came. I was hoping that Patient **F** and Patient **J** did not talk to each other. I did not want to have to explain why one could have an emergency supply and one could not.

The dispenser mentioned that the pharmacist who had worked two days ago had ended up ripping up a patient's prescription after he had become abusive. I was too busy to ask questions about it!

I found the Gabapentin prescription that the Patient **D** had mentioned. It was a week old and had not been dispensed. Oh well!

These issues will be familiar to anyone that works in pharmacy. It is especially difficult for a locum as they have to hope that there are no unresolved issues from the previous day and that the right medicines have been ordered. They also have to hope that any notes that they leave get followed up.

Locums sometimes get a bad press [from me!]. I for one could not do it full-time. I like to know everything that is happening in my pharmacy. I have a newfound respect for locums.

I was driving home after the home delivery and my all-time favourite song 'Wonderwall' came on the Radio. It cheered me up. Then I got a phone call from my branch asking if I could pop in and sort out a couple of problems! AAAARRRRGGGHHH!!!

Just Say No

I really should learn to say 'No' once in a while. It's actually quicker and easier than a yes. I got asked to work on Saturday morning for four hours and said yes. I had not been to this pharmacy in a few years but remembered it to be a pleasant one.

I thought I knew how to get there so I did not use my Sat Nav. When it got to 8.55am and I was lost, I pulled over and turned on the Sat Nav. It was seven minutes away. I arrived at 9.02am very embarrassed and apologised profusely.

I was greeted with chaotic scenes. There were thirty baskets to check from yesterday. I sent a cheeky tweet detailing my findings before getting down to the task at hand. Twenty minutes later, the locum agency rang and said that there was a mix-up and that I had to go to another branch twenty miles away!

I looked at the baskets and weighed it up against the car journey and decided to move branches. I was told not to wait for my replacement. The lady from the locum agency told me that there was already someone at the next pharmacy waiting for me to get there so not to worry about getting there ASAP. So I stopped for a McDonalds breakfast! I jest!

The next pharmacy was forty-five minutes away according to the Sat Nav. I started driving and decided to ring them to let them know how long it would take me. Whilst on the phone, I heard police sirens behind me rapidly approaching. Thankfully they had a more important matter to attend to and did not punish my stupidity.

The pharmacy was the scene of my 'Locums deserve respect' chapter. Thankfully it was a lot nicer this time and less problematic. However, I wish I had said no and stayed in bed.

Liar Liar

Patient: Hi, can I have some co-codamol please?

Mr Dispenser: Is it for you or someone else?

Patient: Me.

Mr Dispenser: Have you had it before?

Patient: Yes.

Mr Dispenser: Recently?

Patient: No.

Mr Dispenser: What pain is it for?

Patient: Back pain. Only thing that works.

Mr Dispenser: It's only for three days use.

Patient: Ok.

Mr Dispenser: Are you on any other medication?

Patient: No.

Mr Dispenser: That means over the counter, prescribed or herbal?

Patient: No.

Mr Dispenser: Don't take any paracetamol with this as it contains paracetamol.

Patient: Yeah, I know.

Mr Dispenser: That's £1.49 please.

Patient: Oh, while I'm here can I pick up my prescription. I ordered it last week. Got no tablets left….

A Missing Prescription

Two days ago, I was at work happily (not really) checking away. I shouted John Smithson's [not his real name] name out. No one answered, I repeated myself. There was still no answer. I carried on checking. Then I realised that a woman had been sat in the waiting area for a very long time. I asked what name she was waiting for. She said John Smith (not his real name) and that she had been waiting for 45 minutes! I assumed that she was absent when I had called out the name and that she had now returned or that she had not heard me.

I did not remember checking a prescription for that name so I looked on the computer. Generally, I forget patient's names but remember medications they are taking. John Smith had last had his prescription dispensed in November. Then I remembered John Smithson's prescription. Is there a chance that we had made the fatal mistake of labelling under the wrong name? It happens unfortunately.

The woman was collecting the prescription for her husband. I dug out the prescription and showed her the reverse asking if it was her signature. She said yes, ending the moment of panic. I told her that this was not the prescription she asked for, possibly breaking patient confidentiality and telling her the name on the prescription and that it was similar. This was wrong. However, I was glad that it was not our mistake. It was the receptionist's. She had given her the wrong prescription...

I marched over to reception and spoke to the receptionist explaining that the woman had been given the wrong prescription. The receptionist was in shock. Claiming she had confirmed the address with the woman before she gave it out. I paused and shrugged my shoulders. I turned over the prescription verifying the credibility of this situation by double-checking if it was his signature. She said it was, as far as she knew. Aware of the growing queue at the pharmacy, I left it for the receptionist to sort out.

I went back to the pharmacy and took delight in telling my staff what had happened. It was not our fault. The woman was quietly waiting for forty-five minutes. She would probably still be there if I had not spoken to her!

Then someone turned up asking for John Smithson's prescription. After confirming the address and drug I handed it to him. My Sherlock Holmes moment was now upon me, I was very puzzled and even more curious. Where was John Smith's prescription and why had the woman signed for John Smithson's?

At our pharmacy, waiting prescriptions are placed in white baskets. I spotted a white basket in the far corner of the dispensary. Gazing at the basket I walked over slowly, and there, was John Smith's prescription! WHAT THE HELL WAS GOING ON?!?!!? I turned it over and compared the signature to John Smithson's. They were not identical but similar. During the second round of questioning, the woman had mentioned the signature was his AS FAR AS SHE KNEW!

The woman returned holding a reprint prescription for John Smith. My pharmacy assistant started talking about finding it, I shushed her. I processed the prescription and apologised for it taking an hour and the woman left.

I decided to shred the original and no-one would be none the wiser. That's before my conscience got the better of me. Telling me I should have been honest with the woman. I decided to apologise to the receptionist. I took that morning's purchase of Galaxy Caramel chocolate over to the receptionist and explained that I had found the prescription. She was a lady about it and was glad that it had been found. She refused the chocolate, but accepted a mutual sense of confusion, as we both pondered on why the woman could not recognise her own signature!

Later I ate my Galaxy bar whilst reflecting on the events. I concluded that 1) Pharmacy is never a dull place and 2) chocolate makes you happy....

Dress to Impress

Pharmacists are professionals and should dress as such. I have only come across a couple of pharmacists that still wear white lab coats at work. The majority wear smart attire.

We are told that it is important for us to look professional so that the patient will be more likely to listen and accept our advice. However, I have seen two GPs who wear jeans in their surgery and the patients don't seem to mind. Whilst I was a student I saw one locum pharmacist wear jeans and another wear a skirt and flip flops.

Some companies make their pharmacist wear a uniform e.g. Tesco. Some hospitals have a no tie and long-sleeve shirt policy or a uniform. This is to minimise infections.

I rarely wear a tie at work and the only people that seem to care are my parents. The quality of my clothes is directly proportional to the amount of food that I spill on me at lunch. Be it Armani or Primani, yoghurt stains on black trousers are hard to explain.

John D'Arcy: What does a pharmacist look like?

I learned early on in my career how difficult it would be telling people that I was a pharmacist. Not long after qualifying I was in a pub in the Lake District with two friends, one a pharmacist who had been at College with me and the other, a chap who owned a garage in Lancashire. The garage owner was a good looking bloke, the sort who always got his girl. On entering the pub he instantly spied two girls who became his prey. He engaged them in conversation, and in time, one of the girls asked him, "What do you do?"

He replied, "I am a pharmacist".

What made him think this would improve his pulling power remains to this day a mystery. However the girls replied to him,

"You're not a pharmacist".

"Why am I not a pharmacist?" he asked.

"Because you don't look like a pharmacist", came the reply.

"So, what does a pharmacist look like?" he enquired.

At this point the girls began studying the amassed throng and their gaze moved clockwise around the bar until they got to me.

"Like him" they said.

Guest Blogs

The views of these guest bloggers do not necessarily represent my views. However, they would not be in this book, if they did not.

Badges by Candy Sartan

If I could offer you only one tip for the future, badges would be it.

The long term benefits of wearing badges have been proved by Area Mangers that customers can complain about you easier, whereas the rest of my advice has no basis more reliable than my own meandering experience…

I will dispense this advice now.

Enjoy the power and beauty of your youth; oh never mind; after six months of working with the public you will be ready to retire.

But trust me, in 20 years you'll look back at photos of yourself and recall in a way you can't grasp now how much possibility lay before you and how fabulous you really looked until the frown lines and eye bags took hold….

You're not as fat as you imagine, but cut down on the Christmas biscuits and chocolates from patients just in case.

Don't worry about the future; or worry, but know that worrying is as effective as trying to solve a dosage query by chewing bubble gum.

The real troubles in your life are apt to be things that never crossed your worried mind; the kind that blindside you at 4pm on some idle Tuesday when you realise you forgot to send the order.

Do one thing every day that scares you like telling the addicts that you forgot to send that order and have now run out of methadone.

Sing, but make sure you have a broadcasting licence.

Don't be reckless with other people's hearts; take extra care when dispensing those lisinopril.

Floss, nobody can take medical advice from a pharmacist when he has lunch in his teeth, they will not hear anything you say they will be too distracted by your mouth.

Don't waste your time on jealousy; sometimes you're ahead, sometimes you're behind...but however many MURs you do, it will never be enough for the powers that be.

Remember the compliments you receive, forget the insults; they are usually from the same people, one week you give them their script in superfast time and you're great, the next week you owe them something and you're the worst pharmacy EVER.

Keep your old invoices; throw away your old biros that have dried out.

Stretch.

Get plenty of calcium, copious amounts of milky tea or coffee.

Be kind to your knees, you'll miss them when they're gone from standing for eight hours a day.

Dance...even if you have nowhere to do it but in your own dispensary.

The days are long and you need to find ways of keeping your spirits up.

Read the directions, know the side effects.

Do NOT read pharmacy magazines, they will only make you feel inadequate.

Get to know your locums, you never know when they'll be gone for good and you'll have to cover your own holidays.

Be nice to your dispensers; they are the best link to a tidy and smoothly running dispensary.

Understand that customers come and go, but for the precious few you should hold on to, they will get older and the amount of items per month will only increase.

Work hard to bridge the gaps in geography with delivery drivers because the older you get, the more you need your prescriptions delivered.

Work for a multiple once, but leave before it makes you hard; work for an independent once, but leave before it makes you soft.

Travel.

Accept certain inalienable truths, prices will rise, GPs will philander, you too will get old, and when you do you'll fantasize that when you were young prices were reasonable, GPs were noble and customers respected their pharmacist.

Respect your staff. Don't expect anyone else to support you. Maybe you have public liability insurance, maybe you have union representation; but you never know when either one might run out.

Don't mess too much with your hair, it doesn't look professional to have a neon blue Mohican in the pharmacy.

Be careful whose advice you buy, but, be patient with those who supply it.

Advice is a form of nostalgia, dispensing it is a way of fishing the past from the disposal, wiping it off, painting over the ugly parts and recycling it for more than it's worth. But trust me on the badges...

Pre-reg by @weeneldo

Pre-reg! It's been going for two weeks! It's busy! My feet hurt!

It's a lot different to my local pharmacy. Much busier, so many new things that I've never seen. We're totally rushed off our feet all day but I can guarantee you it'll be 5.30 before you know it. Here's what my typical day has consisted of so far:

8:30am - Leave house, still putting tie on, eating toast, fixing hair, putting on jumper, tying shoes and brushing teeth at same time. Drive to work singing at top of lungs and steering with feet while I play air drums.

9:00am - Shop opens for business.

9:12am - I arrive for business.

9:15am - Having drank half a bottle of Irn-Bru to let my eyes stay open longer than 4 seconds, I slowly start to print labels and stick them on to the medications for people who get their prescription dispensed in daily/weekly instalments. An important part of this process is repeatedly making an arse of printing the labels, then sticking the labels onto the wrong things.

10:00am - Perform "technical support" by loudly shouting abuse at the computer in front of a small child and her grandmother.

10:01am - Give computer therapeutic massage by smashing keyboard with fists.

10:20pm - Serve a short chain of methadone patients. Somehow get methadone all over hands and counter. Consider selling fingers for "penny-a-lick" but decide against plan after visualising potential Dragon's Den episode in my head.

10:40am - Prepare to dispense "compliance aid" for patient on 17,000 different medicines. Realise that instead of sending us prescriptions, doctor has sent "MEDICASHUNZ PLX" written on a king-size Rizla.

11:10am - Having sourced prescriptions for the patient's medication and popped out millions of tiny tablets into individual compartments by day and time, I knock it all over and cover the floor in pills. I cry.

11:30am - Our orders come in from the pharmaceutical suppliers. Comparing what we've received against the invoice, we soon notice that instead of 20 boxes of Simvastatin 40mg and 10 boxes of Bisoprolol 5mg, they've sent us 3 pints of gold-top and a white loaf.

12:00pm - LUUUUUNCH!!!!!!!!!!!!!!

1:00pm - I return from lunch and get straight back into the action. Prescriptions have been collected from the doctors' surgeries and must be dispensed. The bench soon starts to fill up with more drugs than a Glasgow Christmas.

1:40pm - I'm standing at the bench dispensing. It's confusing. The paracetamol is fighting the ibuprofen and Adrian Chiles just burrowed in through the floor. I realise that I've fallen asleep standing up and have been dreaming for the last 15 minutes.

2:20pm - A nice lady from one of the doctors' surgeries phones. She wants to know if we can help fix her computer. I ask if her computer is made out of tablets. She says no. In that case we can't help.

3:00pm - About this time I start counting down the minutes until the end of the day. Sometimes I even take my watch off to stop me looking at the time every 5 seconds.

3:30pm - A patient gets upset because we never picked up their prescription from the surgery. Of course they didn't actually ask us to pick it up for them, but who likes a pedant?

4:10pm - A razor sharp foil tablet blister pack nearly takes my hand off. In reality it's a 2mm paper cut, but there's enough blood to drown Dappy from N-Dubz.

4:20pm - A patient brings their child into the pharmacy with chickenpox. My brain screams at me: "RUNNNNNN!!!!!". I dive behind the counter and commando-roll into the store-room. I've never had chickenpox before and am I hell getting it now.

5:00pm - Half an hour to go now, so naturally people will start wanting us to, like, help them and that. The BASTARDS. The massive queue of prescriptions along the bench will ensure that future comedians have plenty of material about the length of time a prescription takes in the chemist. I run about fetching tablet boxes, printing off wrong labels. Fixing the labels. Fixing something else on the labels. The computer breaks. I knock over a big pile of stuff. I trip over a stool. I walk into someone. The printer runs out of labels. More Irn-Bru. Finally we clear the last prescription. Steam is pouring out my ears. I sway slightly forwards. I sway slightly backwards.

5:30pm - END OF THE DAY!!! That beautiful trundling sound of the shutters closing behind me. Standing outside, I'm now free. I walk to my car, open the door and collapse in my seat. Bastard! I left my phone in the shop.

Peachy by @weeneldo

sniff

It happened again :(

sniff

The bad lady said things about my bum.

She's a regular patient, and recently she's been following a bit of a routine every Saturday when she comes in. She stands at the counter and goes into a total daze. When Papier, our pharmacist, speaks to the patient to bring her out of it, the patient replies something along the lines of:

"Sorry, but Enzo's got a really nice arse in those trousers. It's like a peach, I could just bite it."

Usually I stand within earshot feeling rather uncomfortable. Well not today. Today, once 'brought round' by Papier, the patient directly addressed me and gladly informed me of what she would do if I was "her man". I had to go round the back and scrub my body clean with Brillo pads and bleach.

It's now reached the stage where every permanent member of staff who has ever worked in our shop has been chatted up by at least one patient. As I hypothesised in work, we must just be a really sexy shop.

On a less sexually objectifying note, today was my second last Saturday as a student in my local pharmacy. I'm still not sure if I'm going to miss the place.

I came to the shop 2 months after I started my degree - way back in 2006. My previous job had been on the tills in McDonald's, so it was like a whole new world I was stepping into. You know that bit in The Shawshank Redemption where the old guy gets let out of prison and can't fit into his new job and his new life on the outside? That's what I was like. Through force of McDonald's habit (and much to the amusement of my new pharmacy colleagues), I always found myself asking to go to the toilet or to take a drink of water. Of course things soon changed and I became the lazy wee bastard I am now.

Breeds of Pharmacists by Candy Sartan

In over a decade of working in pharmacy I've worked with dozens and dozens of pharmacists. Just as David Attenborough lives in the jungles of South America and gets to learn which breed of lizard or spider is which, I have learned the different types of pharmacist, and can even spot a pharmacist out of their own habitat, the pharmacy.

There are three groups of Males: The briefcase, the rucksack and the carrier bag. These are self-explanatory but have specific breed 'standards' if you like, which are particular to each type.

Type 1. The briefcase guy.

This type of pharmacist arrives either on time or early, wearing a suit and with clean shoes. He will be in a BMW car of any age but it will be clean. He may come from a multi-car household though so if he does show up in a Citroen C2, don't be fooled, his wife will have had to borrow the Beemer and he will be forced to drive her car. But, you will be unaware of this as he will park it four streets away to avoid being spotted.

On opening the leather briefcase there will be a plethora of pharmaceutical gubbins. His own BNF, often with pages marked with highlighter or a Post-It hanging out to mark where he's up to. Another tome to be found in the good ole briefcase could be the MEP, always a tantalising read over lunch in the consultation room. A common item in this pharmacist's briefcase is a responsible pharmacist certificate IN COLOUR and perhaps even, yes, laminated. (a far cry from the black and white printable ones on our computer).This pharmacist will bring his own pen. Not just a rep pen or a bic biro. Oh no. We could be looking at a Staedtler or Parker pen, often in its own case or in a set with a matching mechanical pencil.

Now, the briefcase guy can be any age but the older 'BG' will have a well-thumbed copy of the MIMs from as far back as 2003, in case he is checking a nursing home or MDS tray. Along with his MIMs he may carry (and I have seen this) his own pair of plastic tweezers for fishing around in blister packs. This next item never varies. Sandwiches. Wrapped in foil or cling film BG doesn't mind but he has to have sandwiches for lunch and he has to have had them made that morning and placed into an airtight container for later consumption. He may have a yoghurt (Shape is very common as Mrs BG does the weekly shop and buys the bumper pack) BG will bring his own spoon. He is a well prepared chap who doesn't like to chance it that the pharmacy he will be going to will have zero cutlery.

BG will sign in without prompting and have his posh certificate on display before you have got the kettle on. He will have any CD deliveries and supplies written up, if not as they go out, by the end of his shift. He will help any colleague with training whether it be their OTC training, the technician course or a pre-reg needing some guidance. He will have any information in that briefcase and if not he will have found it in the pharmacy within five minutes.

BG has a tidy diary with colour coded entries and an easy reference filing system of useful information. He knows where he is at any given day and knows distances, opening and closing times of every shop he's ever worked in.

Lastly, the locum claim form. He will have a pressed copy of this in his 'locum forms' section and remove it in due course and it will be perfectly filled in and dealt with by the most responsible looking person in that day.

Type 2. The rucksack guy.

This happy-go-lucky pharmacist will be smart looking but without the constraints of a tie. Perhaps he will be wearing a jumper over just a shirt. Elbow pads will not be out of the question. The footwear is a giveaway of RG. Although I can spot him a mile off I don't quite understand the temperature requirements RG has with regards to his footwear. He wears socks with sandals. Now, I am not sure whether the sandals are on first, but it's a little nippy, so he puts the socks on to stop the frost or whether the socks are on first, but in case of overheating he just wears sandals. It may even be a fashion statement I admit I'm baffled by this.

Rucksack guy will be just to say on time. He may even fly through the door dead on opening time. No time will be lost though as he has no jacket to remove, no responsible pharmacist sign to unpack and no formalities like shaking hands. You will just know who he is. He has the rucksack. You may have to ask him to sign in as he is too busy finding the kettle and making himself at home to be bothered with such trifles.

RG will bring his own pen, usually a free rep pen pilfered from the last locum shift or a plain old bic, hell, it may be from the bookies, he isn't fussy in the pen department (or any other department actually). This pen he arrives with will be left in your pharmacy when he leaves. He's a fly-by-night pen collector.

RG has a diary. It is shoved full of bits of paper with phone numbers and bookings, even expenses receipts. He is slightly disorganised but with a little guidance he will have settled in by lunchtime.
His lunch, incidentally is practically all that is in the rucksack. He will have brought a drink, usually a can of coke (iron bru in Scotland), a packet of crisps, a pre-packed sandwich he got at the Tesco petrol station on the way in and perhaps some Dairylea dunkers. RG isn't afraid of being in touch with his inner schoolboy, in fact, now you come to mention it, this could be the hidden meaning behind his style.

He will ask you for a claim form, he won't have one with him, the only other thing in the rucksack is probably a John Grisham book, to read at lunchtime, if he gets bored.

Type 3. Carrier bag guy.

Where to start with CBG. We have all worked with one, he is firstly, obviously a CBG by his notable absence ten minutes after his shift was due to start. Not even organised enough to have noted down the phone number of the branch and call to say he's late you know you're going to be in for a day of total chaos.

CBG may appear any time after he is expected so be on the lookout. He will breeze through the door past disgruntled patients waiting outside looking with daggers and remain oblivious to the awkward conversations we've had to have. "But my prescription is only there, I brought it in yesterday. I can practically see it on the shelf" then as if some magic force field has been lifted, people can now be given what was only 6 feet away from them all the time.

CBG could be wearing anything. Usually, however whatever he is wearing he will have worn yesterday, and possibly the day before that. His hair will be messy, but not in the stylish "just stepped out of the salon" way, in the "I only got out of bed 20 minutes ago" way.

CBG has brought very little with him. No pen, no lunch, no certificate, no claim form and no diary. He may not even have a diary. I have worked with a CBG who literally had everything he needed to know, written on scraps of paper. CBG's mind is total chaos. He will drive a banger. If you were to look in the car you would find a representation of CBG's brain. Empty wrappers, old newspapers, maybe the odd hobo that sneaked in there.

This is your fly by the seat of your pants kind of pharmacist. Lunchtime comes and he asks directions to the nearest shop, gathers all the loose change from his pockets (probably found on the floor of old betsy the car) and nips out for what he promises will be 10 minutes. 35 minutes later he still has not returned. CBG of course doesn't wear a watch. The end of the day approaches and he still hasn't signed in and there's a pile of CD scripts and invoices to enter. He probably won't ask you for a claim form because he forgets, he still hasn't submitted last month's ones yet.

Obviously, new pharmacists are produced every year from the production line and over the years, what with GM crops and natural selection, some variances may occur but these are your three basic types of male pharmacist. No offence is meant to any pharmacist, whether he be a straight-laced BG or a flighty CBG. These are just my observations over the years. But boy, are they accurate!

I Have A Smart Phone! by @ApothecaryTales

Remember folks, just because you have a smart phone, it doesn't make you smart!

I have lots of patience...LOTS! You have to, in the wonderful-almost-seems-imaginary world of retail pharmacy. It's uber tough working out there, especially with what seems to be an increased population of idiots that makes up the majority of society nowadays. I DO NOT however have patience with fools that have no grasp of the English language. Now, before you jump all over me, I am not talking about people with English as a second language. I am talking about those morons with their moron parents and moron grandparents who can't even put six words together to make a comprehensible sentence. I am talking about the ones who dropped out of kindergarten and get confused at the L-M-N-O-P part of the Alphabet song. The ones that can't count to 512 but recognize what the characters look like on a pill. Now it's bad enough when they are stupid right in front of your face but for me at least, I get more irritated when it's on the phone.

Not sure about the rest of you, but I hate the phone. Unless it's a new prescription being called in I usually don't have time to shoot the shit with you over the phone for three minutes while you are yelling at your kid in the background...GET LOST! If I ask you a question, do not answer with the following, "Well you see...my kid...eats a bath...and there is corn...and the car fought the pretzel...and I got reports of things...and I ate...and yeah refill it...and diarrhoea happened...and then the Hamburglar"... HUH?...Exactly!

Someone needs to teach these people proper phone etiquette. It's not enough that you have a slow-talking computerized voice giving you prompts on the phone when you call the pharmacy. It's not! If the prompt says dial 1 if you are a prescriber, DON'T DIAL 1 IF YOU AREN'T A FLAMING PRESCRIBER! If the prompt says dial 2 to leave a message, DON'T DIAL 2 AND START PUNCHING IN FLAMING NUMBERS! Cause this will lead me to have to answer my message line just to hear the beeping of numbers. I don't like wasting my time on nonsense! If the prompt says dial 3 to enter your refill numbers, DON'T DIAL 3 AND START TALKING AND THEN CALL ME BACK TELLING ME YOU TRIED CALLING IN REFILLS BUT THE PHONE DIDN'T UNDERSTAND YOU...NO SHIT YOU MORON!

I think you can determine a patient's drug compliance based on how they speak over the phone and what prompts they hit to get to you. If they hit the prescriber line and they aren't a prescriber, or did any of the other things mentioned above, they obviously don't follow directions well and clearly would not be able to understand a prednisone taper typed out for them.

WHEN I PICK UP THE PHONE I SAY, "PHARMACY, HOW MAY I HELP YOU?"

Do NOT be silent for more than 2 seconds, I WILL HANG UP ON YOU!

Do NOT continue a conversation you were having with your baby daddy regarding your unpaid car note and broken XBox, I WILL HANG UP ON YOU!

Do NOT have the first words you say, "Is my prescription ready?"...WHO ARE YOU? GIVE ME A NAME? I give you 2 seconds to continue your sentence and if no name is mentioned I HANG UP ON YOU!

Do NOT tell me to HOLD ON as soon as I pick up... cause guess what? I WILL HANG UP ON YOU!

Do NOT ask me if I have Maxwell House coffee on sale today...not my job! I WILL HANG UP ON YOU!

Do NOT call me and ask for the phone number at the pharmacy down the road I WILL HANG UP ON YOU!

Do NOT call me asking for cash prices on #180 Oxycodone 30mg, I WILL KEEP YOU ON HOLD FOR 5 MINUTES! and then HANG UP ON YOU!

Basically, what I am trying to say is, DON'T CALL ME!

I hate people!

A view from the other side of the counter by @optforoptimism

I try my very hardest to avoid going to the GPs' surgery for three reasons;

1) I hate waiting 40 minutes after my appointment to "get in".

2) I like to think that I don't abuse the service, and therefore try not to go.

3) I hate The Pharmacy afterwards.

The last time I visited the GP was about a year ago. I was almost 8 months pregnant and had a horrific chest infection. Every time I coughed I would pee. Sexy, I know. However, the GP was more concerned about me triggering early labour, so he kindly prescribed me an inhaler.

My local surgery is a new build, with flat screens and comfy chairs; it also has a Lloyds Pharmacy attached to it. Rather than move my car, I tend to wander into it straight from the surgery. My visit to The Pharmacy went like this;

Enter pharmacy. Join the queue and wait for ten years while the Busy Body Counter Lady finishes her conversation about Jim from Bush Street and his bad foot. Further discusses patient information. Asks after grandchildren. Falters to find any new topic to discuss, and beckons me over.

I hand her my prescription (which is free in Wales). I attempt to tear the back off. Very difficult when you have other "waitees" literally sat on the counter between the rack of throat sweets and lip balms and you can't raise your elbows without smacking them in the jaw. I presume they think their prescription will arrive quicker if they invade innocent peoples' personal space.

I hold my breath, not wanting to catch the flu or other disease. Now it's The Wait. You know, the ridiculous amount of time it takes to get a simple prescription filled. I wander about, trying not to stare at badly behaved feral children and their screeching parents. Look at the make-up display. Read a few leaflets on diabetes and heart disease. Avoid the automatic door, if it opens, you see, everyone turns around and glares at you. I play a game of "guess the ailment" but can never truly win, unless Busy Body Counter Lady feels the need to discuss said ailment with patient of my choice.

Stare at a few people going in and out of the Consultancy Room, wondering if they're after the morning after pill or weight-loss tablets. Lose the will to live.

Pick up a packet of Berocca and decided RIGHT THERE AND THEN to start living healthier and taking vitamins for the rest of my life.

Join the queue and wait for ten years while the Busy Body Counter Lady finishes her conversation about Jane from Meyrick Street and her husband's gimpy leg.

I, almost triumphantly, hand over the Berocca and pay by debit card. Decline a bag as they're 5 pence in Wales and I have no change. Wait for a moment longer than I should in case Busy Body Counter lady turns around with a winning smile and says;

"Sophie? Here you are" and hands me a green bag.

She doesn't. I turn and back away, there's no waiting space near the queue or the counter, as the other "waitees" are still lounging on the displays trying to peer into the back. I wander over the knee supports, and before I decide to make the fatal decision to start up running, I stand back in the queue.

And wait for ten years while Busy Body Counter Lady insists on sticking reduced stickers on every single hair dye in the box on the counter. I couldn't count them all but I'd say there was at least fifty thousand.

It's finally my turn and the conversation goes a little something like this;

Me: Shall I just come back another time?

BBCL: What is it you're waiting for?

Me: Well, my prescription (?!)

BBCL: Well what was it for?

Me: Erm, well *CUE Waitees to prick their ears up* nothing exciting...just an inhaler.

BBCL: Well The Pharmacist is going as fast as he can, isn't he Sandra?

Sandra stocking the knee supports nods her head in agreement

Me: Right well, yes, but that isn't what I asked...shall I just come back?

The Pharmacist enters The Pharmacy through the automatic doors, and in true form to the waitees I turn around and glare. His mouth is full of sandwich, with crumbs on his tie and clutching his car keys.

Busy Body Counter Lady has moved on to the next customer.

I have a violent coughing fit and pee myself a little bit.

Lose the will to live and go home.

Isaiah was born a week early.

Now I LOVE the fact that the NHS is free and accessible. I have private cover and wish I could see a GP on that to avoid taking up space in an undervalued commodity. That said, if I had to see a Pharmacist I'd rather just get ill. And die. Ok, that last bit was a bit extreme. Pharmacists have their place and do an excellent job;

Me: What is this? (Opens mouth and allows stranger to peer in)

Pharmacist: Ulcer, go and buy XYZ.

Excellent, what's not to like? But when you are waiting for a script it's like waiting to DIE. Long and unnecessary. EVEN for the stuff they don't have to count. Like an inhaler, for a random, related example.

Next time I have to go, I shall take my baby and my toddler. And feed them Skittles in the waiting room. Let's see how long I'll have to wait THEN.

Disclaimer: I totally love Pharmacists. This, while a TRUE account, was written tongue-in-cheek. Before you come after me with flamed torches, and I end up having to go and get burn relief from erm The Pharmacy

On-call by @navinsewak

On a number of occasions there were 'discussions' between junior pharmacists and junior doctors. Almost all the time these discussions were amicable and involved a 'what do you think, no what do you think?' type of interaction on the phone. Often I got the feeling that this type of discussion, between two highly trained, and clever professionals was in fact an 'I have no-idea what I'm doing, please help me' type of conversation! It would have bit comical (and a good idea for a sit-com) had it not been the case that we were talking about real people, and sometimes life or death situations...

One of the great skills of an on-call pharmacist in a busy London teaching hospital is known as 'juggling'. Juggling the phone, the bleep, annoying nurses at the hatch, and your constantly increasing workload (I was the unlucky resident - dealing with 200 calls a night). It did not matter when patients turned up at the hatch. On one particular night this patient knocked on the pharmacy hatch at 3am in the morning. I cursed under my breath and went to answer the call.

I looked at the patient and said 'can I help you?'.

He gave me the look of 'what took you so long to answer?' and was prompted to utter two words : 'my lips'.

I said 'what about them?'.

He said 'they are dry. Do you have any Vaseline?'

I simply starred at him for what seemed like ages.

He interrupted my gaze with 'Are you listening?'

'Where have you come from?' I said.

'I spent two hours waiting in A&E and they sent me here' he said.

Meanwhile my bleep was going off and I had to keep silencing it.

'Do you have any Vaseline?' he repeated.

Without saying anything, I closed the hatch and went to the pharmacy robot and took out some E45 cream.

'I only have this' I said.

'How much is it?' he said

'£3.29'

'A bit expensive, do you have anything cheaper?' he exclaimed.

'Not at 3am in the morning I don't' I snapped.

'Think I'll leave it he said - I don't want to pay that kind of money' he said.

I gave him a look of disgust as he wandered off.

I went back to my never-ending nightmare of a night to answer the 20 bleeps I'd missed.

Needless to say I wasn't in the best mood!

Pop Culture

These blogs involve The Fresh Prince, game shows, movie gangsters, Fight Club and songs.

Fresh Pharmacist of Bel-Air

Now this is the story all about how

My life got flipped, turned upside down

And I'd like to take a minute just sit right there

I'll tell you how I became the pharmacist of a town called
Bel-Air

In West Yorkshire PCT born and raised

In the dispensary where I spent most of my days

Chilling out, dispensing, relaxing all cool

And all doing some chlamydia screening outside of the
school

When a couple of GPs who were up to no good'

Started making trouble in my neighbourhood

I got in one little fight and my Area manager got scared

And said 'you're moving with your cluster manager in Bel-Air'

I begged and pleaded with her the other day

But she packed my MDS and sent me on my way

She gave me a kissin' and she gave me my ticket

I put my iPod on and said I might as well kick it

I whistled for a delivery driver and when it came near

The License plate said 'Fresh' and had a pestle 'n' mortar in the mirror

If anything I could say that this delivery van was rare

But I thought now forget it, yo home to Bel-Air

I pulled up to a pharmacy about seven or eight

And I yelled to the delivery driver 'Yo, home smell you later'

Looked at my pharmacy I was finally there

To sit on my throne as the pharmacist of Bel-Air

If Pharmacy was a game show

Have I got news for you: Rival multiples led by their Area Managers as team captains make fun of the week's pharmacy news.

Mastermind: This replaces CPD entries.

Catchphrase: An illegible prescription is presented and pharmacists are asked to say what they see.

The Generation game: A ten item prescription is flashed on screen for 10 seconds and then they have to dispense it correctly.

Blankety Blank: A crucial detail is missed off a prescription and pharmacists are asked to guess

Telly Addicts: Staff members discuss last night's TV

Million pound drop live: Patients start off with a hundred tablets and gamble them by answering questions on their medication. This replaces MURs.

So you think you can dispense?: If you make a near miss, you are fired. Last one standing gets to keep their job.

Masterchef: Technicians extemporaneously dispense items with points for colour, taste, texture and efficacy.

University Challenge: Pharmacy students from different universities compete to see which is the best university.

Weakest Link: Instead of the pre-registration exam, students are put under pressure to answer questions.

Family Fortunes: Two families both on benefits compete. 'We asked 100 people to name what they tick on the back of their prescription….'

Would I lie to you?: The host asks patients to give medication histories and addicts to tell us why they missed yesterday's collection.

Gladiators: The age old battle of Pharmacists Versus GPs but with lycra

@Cocksparra: The Krypton Factor. Trying to fit soluble paracetamol into the only tablet cartons you have left

Gangster

You may be surprised by how being a pharmacist is a lot like being a gangster. Below are gangster terms but they seem very familiar:

Boss: Sometimes referred to as Father, Godfather or Uncle in the old tradition, the boss is the leader of the Mafia Family = **Superintendent**

Capo: Originally referred to a Mafia boss but in more recent usage refers to a minor leader within a Mafia family, chief of a crew. Also referred to as a captain, skipper or lieutenant = **Area Manager**

Consigliere: A translation of this word as "counsellor" has led to a mistaken impression about the position's duties (that the consigliere is an adviser to the boss). Actually, the consigliere post is intended to serve the family membership, by granting a channel of communication to the boss = **Head of Professional Standards**

Cosa Nostra: To many, this is the proper name of the Mafia in the United States. In fact, it was an effort by some mob bosses to refer to their shared secret society WITHOUT naming it. The phrase translates to, "our thing." = **GPhC**

Made: Formally inducted into the Mafia through a ceremony. Prospective members are called to a meeting without being given a reason. Through an elaborate ritual, they are then invited to join the Mafia. They are typically told the rules of the society, its history and hierarchy, and the general disciplinary measure for disobedience – death = **passing the pre-registration exam**

Muscle: Intimidate. Also those who function as underworld thugs = **Technicians**

Muscle in: Invade a rival's racket or territory through force = **100 hour pharmacy**

Shake down: Obtain money or other concessions from businesses or individuals by using intimidation or extortion = **Prescription charge**

Wiseguy: A "made" member of a Mafia organization = **Pharmacist**

These are quotes from gangster movies that relate to pharmacy:

"Never tell anyone outside the Family what you are thinking again." (Vito (Don) Corleone, Godfather) = Patient confidentiality is important.

"Keep your friends close, but your enemies closer". (Micheal Corleone, Godfather Part II) = You may not like the people you work with.

"Just when I thought I was out… they pull me back in." (Michael Corleone, Godfather Part III) = This happens when you need the toilet and a patient wants to talk to you.

"The entire British Empire was built on cups of tea, and if you think I'm going to war without one, mate, you're mistaken." (Eddie, Lock, Stock and Two Smoking Barrels) = Substitute war with work and it makes sense.

"As far back as I can remember I always wanted to be a gangster." (Henry Hill, Goodfellas) = Work experience in pharmacy as a teenager is important.

"If my answers frighten you then you should cease asking scary questions" (Jules, Pulp Fiction) = Look mate, all I asked was if you were taking any other medication!?!

"That's thirty minutes away. I'll be there in ten." (The Wolf, Pulp Fiction) = Sadly not a mantra deployed by locums.

"Say hello to my little friend!" (Tony Montana, Scarface) = Have you met Susan, our new short dispenser?

Yours sincerely,

The Wiseguy with great Muscle

The Rules of Pharmacy Club

There are many rules in pharmacy. These can be found in your standard operating procedures. However, evidence has come to light about an unofficial but very important set of rules:

1] You do not talk about patients outside the pharmacy.

2] You do NOT talk about patients outside the pharmacy, except on Twitter.

3] If someone says 'stop' or the inspector visits, the pharmacy is over.

4] Only two guys maximum should work at any one pharmacy. Any more is unnatural.

5] Only deal with one patient at a time. Wait in line!

6] No white coats, no trainers.

7] Inappropriate conversations in the pharmacy will go on for as long as they have to.

8] If this is your first time at PHARMACY CLUB, you have to put the kettle on.

Songs about Pharmacy

These song titles could easily have been about pharmacy.

One Direction: What Makes You Beautiful: Our make-up

Olly Murs ft Rizzle Kicks: Heart Skips A Beat: Atrial Fibrillation

Bruno Mars: The Lazy Song: Some locums

Cee Lo Green: Forget You: Nasty customers

Black Eyed Peas: I Gotta Feeling: How patients describe their symptoms

Aretha Franklin: "Respect" This is what we want from GPs

Beatles: "Help!": Referring to the pharmacist

All Shook Up: Elvis Presley: Antibiotic spills

My Name Is: Eminem: Patients ordering their repeat medicines

Celine Dion :"My Heart Will Go On (Love Theme From 'Titanic')": Only if you comply

Backstreet Boys: "I Want It That Way": Fussy patients

MC Hammer : "U Can't Touch This": P meds

Nelly: Hot In Here: Team Menopause

The Killers: Somebody Told Me: Pharmacy gossip

@helenroot: Oops I did it again - Britney Spears. (Sunday morning EHC PGD)

@helenroot: The Drugs don't work - The Verve. (MUR hell)

@helenroot: Constant Craving: KD Lang: Biscuits. The dispenser's diet will start tomorrow

You're the pharmacy that I want

D= Boy/ Danny

G=Girl/Sandy

B: both

G: Tell me about it stud!

The new counter assistant is hot

B: I got chills, they're multiplyin'.

I have flu like symptoms

And I'm losin' control.

I have diarrhoea

'Cause the power you're supplyin',

My tens machine is on..

It's electrifyin'

Too high a setting

G: You better shape up,

I expect great advice

'cause I need a man

I can't get the top off the methadone bottle

and my heart is set on you.

No other option available to me

You better shape up;

I expect the branded stuff

You better understand

My auntie has medical training so I know what I want

To my heart I must be true.

I love honesty

B: Nothin' left, nothin' left for me to do.

I am currently out of work

Both: You're the one that I want.

Boots is shut

(you are the one I want), o,o, oo, honey.

Otherwise I would go there

The one that I want.

I can't see a doctor for two weeks

(you are the one I want), o,o,oo, honey.

Otherwise I would go there

The one that I want

The wait at the walk-in centre is too long

(you are the one i want want), o,o, ooooo

I hate you

The one I need.

I'm desperate

Oh, yes indeed.

Maybe

G: If you're filled with affection,

You need to lose weight

You're too shy to convey,

Speak up child!

Meditate in my direction.

Don't come near me

Feel your way.

Don't touch me

B: I better shape up, 'cause you need a man

I must do some CPD

G: I need a man who can keep me satisfied.

I wish all medicines came in chocolate flavour

B: I better shape up if I'm gonna prove

Do tweets count as CPD?

G: you better prove that my faith is justified.

Otherwise I will contact that PCT thingy

B: Are you sure?

Anything else I can help you with?

Both: Yes, I'm sure down deep inside.

No

Both: You're the one that I want.

Boots is shut

(you are the one i want), o,o, oo, honey.

Otherwise I would go there

The one that I want.

I can't see a doctor for two weeks

(you are the one i want want), o,o,oo, honey.

Otherwise I would go there

The one that I want

The wait at the walk-in centre is too long

(you are the one i want want), o,o, ooooo

I hate you

The one I need.

I'm desperate

Oh, yes indeed.

Maybe

Anecdotes

These were sent to be my various people in different countries via email, Twitter, FB and LinkedIn.

Hospital

@jonathanmason

My friend was doing his pre-reg in a hospital pharmacy department and had to talk to a patient about his suppositories. He sat down with the patient and explained what they were for and how to use them – carefully explaining that he should take a suppository out of its wrapper and then insert it into his rectum.

"My what?"

"Your rectum"

"What?"

"Insert it into your anus"

"Huh"

"Erm, push it into your back passage"

"Eh? Are you telling me to shove it up my arse?"

"Yes"

"Well, why didn't you say so in the first place?"

I was in charge of the dispensary last Wednesday morning. One of our new doctors came to ask if she could get an emergency supply of her contraceptive pill. She lived in Nottingham and had forgotten to book an appointment to see her GP for a new supply & she had now run out. I told her that we only dispensed emergency supplies for doctors for items that would keep them in work, ie antibiotics, reliever inhalers, and the like.

She told me that a supply from us WOULD keep her in work because otherwise she would have to take the afternoon off to go & see her GP, and that it WAS an emergency because if she got pregnant she would then be off work for months! I told her that there were 'other ways' to not get pregnant - to which she replied (quite seriously) "Well what are they then, because I don't know of any?" I fear for her patients.

I hope everyone is well this August, because it's a bad time to be ill! The new doctors have started:

How about Haloperidol 50mg once daily? That ought to calm them down!

Or sleeping tablets prescribed at 8am? That's just cruel.

And lastly: Thromboprophylaxis - 4500 units s/c daily. Care to tell me the drug name or are we just guessing now?

Trevor Jenkins

After a couple of years of experience at SGH: Dr W, Consultant Physician of the very old school, with the driest of humour, wrote prescriptions resembling ECG traces more than "Prescribing". Once used to interpreting the most difficult prescriptions, I did good trade with junior Doctors, especially surgeons getting Dr W's referrals (paid out in pints in the hospital social club), interpreting his medical notes. One day Dr W came into the Pharmacy with a patient's medical record notes and asked for me by name. Adrenergic surge!

"Yes Dr W?"

Dr W: "I wonder if you could read what I have written here please . . . .?"

So I did!

@spikynorman

Phone call one Sunday about a patient who had put a diclofenac suppository in the wrong orifice (if I tell you she was a she, you should be able to guess!) They wanted to know if it could cause any damage.

Patient turned up and asked for a word "in confidence". She'd been sold a Canesten pessary the day before but she complained it had hurt and was "ever so uncomfortable". She wanted to complain to the company. On questioning it turned out she hadn't taken the wrapper off first!

@mumgonecrazy

It was my first day as a pre-reg. My very first day. I arrived early wearing brand new trousers and a lovely blouse. I had new socks and shoes on. It was like the first day I school. I was issued a regulation white lab coat (they used to be all the rage!). I was taken on a tour of the hospital. It was probably about 9:30. I had been in my new place of work precisely one hour. A&E was next on the list of places to visit.

Now remember it was August. It had been a lovely summer. I had worn shorts and T-shirt all July. I hadn't anticipated on the heat from being fully clothed, and then the addition of a lab coat was just too much.

A lovely pharmacy technician called Pam took me into one of the treatment rooms. There was no one there but us. She was showing me the stock cupboards.........it was all too much......... Pam did her best to catch me! That's right! I fainted. Passed out cold!!

I woke up to find Pam holding my legs in the air (thank heavens I was wearing trousers!) A nurse heard all the kerfuffle and ran for a doctor. A doctor looked in and asked "Are you okay?"

"Yes!" was my reply. And he left me. Lying there on the floor! I was helped to a bed and lay there for 15 minutes before being taken back to pharmacy for a cup of tea. That was the first day!

Many years ago, when team spirit and camaraderie were valued, a junior pharmacist was working a spring Saturday shift at her district general. She received a call: A patient was being transferred back from the regional tertiary care centre to the local ICU.

This patient Alan Peter Rilfool, had major issues still to be resolved in terms of metabolic imbalance and epilepsy control whilst being nil-by-mouth due to major gut surgery.

The junior pharmacist spent an hour calculating the adaptations required for parenteral nutrition and trying to source complex epilepsy drugs. Finally, she accepted defeat and contacted her senior.

The senior pharmacist, close friend of the ICU team, checked the name of Mr A.P.Ril-fool.

American Pharmacy

If you thought that crazy things only happened to us Brits, then you would be mistaken. My comments are in bold.

@Wojciethromycin

"What can I put on my ear? I nicked it with a chainsaw"...do I even want to know how this came about?

I've not had a chainsaw related consultation yet, but it's still early in the day.

I had to deal with a patient that swallowed $500 in cash today...long story.

I hope it wasn't in coins!

@RxLauren

Explain the phenomenon in the pharmacy with people walking in with canes & then leaving them in the store? How far do they get?

They get quite far in my experience. They normally sprint back to collect it.

Woman came to the drive through to ask if she could take her BP. I said I didn't think her arm would fit through the window. I wish I was kidding.

I once saw a website for an internet pharmacy who were apparently offering flu vaccinations.

You know the conversation is going to be interesting when a patient starts it with, "I have this weird rash on my groin area

Been there too. I had managed to block out the mental images with hypnosis until now!

"what do you do for a living?" Stand.

The only time I get to sit down is on the toilet.

"I'll pick it up this afternoon - around 11." Afternoon = after 12.

I struggle with the morning/afternoon dilemma when answering the phone.

Referring to drugs in their brand names. I like to confuse customers on purpose.

Referring to simvastatin as a HMG CoA reductase inhibitor also works.

I love it when patients comment on how busy we are then continue to make our job harder.

Patients were placed on this earth to trouble their pharmacists.

We come in early to get ahead. We don't come in early to open early.

I come in early to catch up from yesterday!

That patient that you do something for, so from then on they will only talk to you because they think anyone else will mess up.

Giving them the name of another member of staff is the best thing.

Wife calls all over city to find Cialis for husband. He's going out of town and "he has to have it!" She doesn't know what Cialis is.

I wish Mrs Dispenser was that helpful.

I wonder when I'll see one of my customers faces flash across the screen while I watch the late news.

I wonder that about some of the doctors too.

Lauren

A lady had a prescription for Percocet (oxycodone and paracetamol combination), with directions to "Take 1/2 to 1 tablet every 4 to 6 hours as needed for pain." This Einsteinette asked, "How will I know which half has the oxycodone in it?"

She needs to know which half to sell!

What to say? We are all familiar with the customer who comes in and decides to vent all of his frustrations upon us. Well, there I was, with one technician (who by the way was an ex-career marine), when this big mouth came in and vented. He managed to heap one expletive upon another until I could listen no more. So, I used that old saying, "If I wanted to hear from an asshole, I'd fart". My tech froze; the customer turned scarlet from anger, and I knew this guy was coming over the counter for me. The tech whispered something to him and he turned and left the premises. By the way -- the next day he was back, apologizing.

I will only employ technicians with military experience from now on.

@RxLauren

When my friend dates a new guy she takes a picture of his meds in his med cabinet & asks me if he's safe. It's one of the perks of having pharmacist friends.

Finding EHC/Plan B in there would be worrying!

@RPHTOTHESTARS

"My friend says I need a vitamin, what do I take?"

"What for?"

" I don't know, you're the pharmacist"

The most expensive one.

"I need to buy something that begins with the letter B. No, I don't know what it's for. I thought that was the pharmacist's job"

Bra?

@*pokey_pineapple*

This should tell you something. The pharmacist (she's a regular here) didn't know if this store has a vacuum. They do!

Are we supposed to clean?

@*RxSchoolProbs*

I've been here 2 years... who the hell is this kid in front of me?

Very true. Attending lectures appears to be a hobby.

@*SaraMac22*

Does anyone else feel extremely awkward while shaking up two bottles of antibiotics at the same time. It looks so bad!!

Yes.

I love hearing drug commercials and knowing what they are talking about!

To be fair, the drug commercials don't even know what they are talking about!

The patient's guide to pharmacy things not to be done

This thread appeared on the Pharmacy Forum website. Some of the comments appear in other chapters in the book.

Sir_Dispensalot

Feel free to try to attempt to barge your way past the pharmacist as he shuts the shop door, key in the lock and with the alarm on countdown, after all with all that going on, the shop must surely be open. The staff will be more than pleased to cancel the alarm, ring the security company to tell them not to send the police out for a double alarm activation and process your script which you possessed for over a week.

Weenoldo

Tell the pharmacist you can't swallow normal paracetamol tablets and must have caplets, but happily take your metformin 850mg.

Ickle_nymph

Screech at the pharmacist "Are you even a real pharmacist!?" after being told something you don't want to hear. I was witness to that not so long ago, and the whole thing actually amused me. We now rib that particular pharmacist when anything goes wrong and tell him "It's alright, you're not a real pharmacist anyway."

Lillylemon

Arrive at 9.30 in the morning to collect your owing which you were told would be ready after 12 noon and complain because the delivery has not arrived. If you are late and do not arrive until 10.30 insist that the dispenser searches through the 15 large boxes for that one bottle of eye drops.

Nik

Bring in a veterinary CD script and expect it to be dispensed on the day, preferably within 5 minutes. It's a pharmacy - they should have these things in, right ?

SolomonQ

Ask for an emergency supply because you forgot to order your prescription, which the pharmacist agrees to do, but sulk and give out sighs of unrest when it takes longer than two minutes, the three patients waiting before you obviously don't need their medication as much as you even though they've bothered to get a prescription.

DispenserJosh

Fail to read the massive sign on the counter you have been staring at for 30 mins stating that the pharmacist is on lunch.

Shout abuse at the pharmacist when they come back, after all, they don't need to eat like normal human beings??

Walk around the front counter clearly separating the dispensary from the shop floor. Look confused when you realise all the people in white coats have stopped what they are doing and are looking at you, one of them then says "sorry, do you mind waiting with the other customers?"

Pharmanaut

Always test-fire your inhaler at random intervals (or during the adverts on TV) to make sure it is still working.

If anything bad has happened to you in the last 25 years and you want an apology for it, make sure you tell the pharmacist.

Swearing at the pharmacist is compulsory. Make sure you learn a new expletive for each visit as it shows how clever you are.

Never say "please" or "thank you" they are unnecessary words and take too much time to use.

A customer was knocking on the door for half-an-hour, looking up at stock-room window shouting. We had left the light on in the stock room and someone thought that we all lived in the "flat above".

Go in and complain about everything even if it is not related to pharmacy, and expect everyone to stop work to listen and sympathise. Example; constant phone calls from double glazing salesmen, junk mail etc.

Feel like saying... 'Just sign this disclaimer saying that I attempted to do my job properly but you refused to let me'

Tell the pharmacist that they should refund the coach trip you missed because the patient information leaflet said avoid exposure to sunlight

Defblade

Come in 3 days in a row asking for your repeat script from the surgery; contact the surgery who contact the pharmacy as the script has been done... but not arrived. On the 3rd day of chasing, say "oh, by the way, do you need this green bit of paper at all?" and unfold it from your wallet.

Toilet Humour

Some people scratch their head, when they see or hear that someone else has head lice, so when they see someone with threadworm or pubic lice, do they....?

I went for a quick wee as the pharmacy was empty. I came back and there were 8 people waiting. I must wee quicker. I may be institutionalised. Also would like not to have to announce to everyone that I am going to the toilet in case they sell a box of 32 paracetamol!

Knocking on the door while I'm having a wee to tell me to hurry up as there are patients waiting doesn't help. I can't do it under pressure.

The main reason I became a pharmacist is so that I can advise my mate via text about his rash down below.

Helen Root

"I'll just fetch the Pharmacist". It's those fail safe words that all counter assistants, dispensers and Pre-reg pharmacists use. Go on, admit, it-you miss being able to ask the Pharmacist some days. So, it was one afternoon when I spotted my counter assistant with two oriental looking customers over by the shelves with the haemorrhoid treatments. Here we go I thought. There was lots of pointing and confused looks and then the inevitable, "I'll just fetch the Pharmacist". When I asked my counter assistant what they wanted, she said she want sure and they didn't speak much English.

So, over I walk to two young ladies with a crumpled piece of paper looking confused. The only word they said to me was 'no toilet' and showed me a piece of paper with the word Anusol on it. Brilliant, they either have piles or are constipated. How the heck do I establish this? Since my Chinese was a little on the poor side.

I decided that since trying to describe piles was the more difficult of the two options, decided to go for the constipation option. I said "no toilet" and they nodded and then I pointed to my bottom and they nodded. Then I thought, nothing else for it, what word will they understand, obviously "stool" wasn't an option. So I decided in "poo". I also then slipped into the typical Brit abroad syndrome (say it in English, but loudly) and started saying "no, poo?" and repeating it louder and louder. I could hear the girls sniggering in the dispensary and knew I sounded stupid. However, the word Poo, was exactly what the issue was and the patient was then very happy when I showed them some senna. Needless to say, once they had left the store, the staff when rolling about at me shouting "poo" very loudly in the shop.

Abs

It was lunchtime at my old workplace in a beauty chain that has a few pharmacies and though it was busy, I had to 'go'. I whispered to my counter assistant and rushed upstairs to the toilet. When I came back I got to hear the tail-end of a conversation that apparently went a little like this:

'I'm sorry madam but I can't give you your prescription until the pharmacist gets back'.

'Well I need to go back to work'.

I'm sorry but you'll have to wait'.

'Well that's just not good enough! Where is she'?

The part I got to hear was 'She had to go to the toilet, I'm sure she'll be back soon'.

'Well I'm in a hurry can't you page her?'

Trevor Jenkins

A stunning blonde shapely young female patient arrived in the deserted Pharmacy waiting room, and always looking for work I announced I would be dealing with this lady! She presented the unmistakeable GUM (Genito-Urinary Medicine) script, with Deteclo prescribed. Heart-sink for me and polite knowing grins from all staff. Counselling the patient with instructions and side-effects, she picked them up, looked them over and said " Oh, they weren't like this last time!" What to say? With a lovely smile while looking into my eyes, she breathed a polite "thanks" and she went. When she was out of sight, I turned, to a circle of staff crying with laughter!

Cameron Kinnell

This old boy comes in one day asking for something for worms in his dog. "What sort of worms", said I. He goes into his pocket pulls out a matchbox opens it and it's full of dog shit and worms.

Stephen Riley

Whilst serving a female customer, my partner was discussing with her what she wanted. It was treatment for crabs for her husband. She said "He is a long distance lorry driver and he gave a lift to someone and then got them as the person must have been a bit unclean and left them on the seat".

@Checkedshoes

It is the season of burnt sausages and badly cooked chicken. Or as pharmacist's call it, Imodium Season.

@lolaskates

When we had senna liquid out of stock, a man came in. He was a regular patient.

'How are you sir?

'Not very well'

'Sorry to hear that Sir. What's wrong?'

'I haven't had a decent shit since October!

Pharmanaut

Because the staff in the pharmacy are not human, you can complain to the NHS if they take a few minutes to go to the toilet. It only takes a few minutes to complain to cause days of disruption to the pharmacy with monitoring visits. Be sure not to ring the PCT at lunchtime though.

Joanna H

One day, Heather was asked to measure this lady for compression hosiery. She came back from the consultation room and said "Never, ever, ever, ever again!!!", we all looked at her and asked what happened. This lady farted whilst being measured by Heather and pretended that nothing happened. No apology, no "oops!" or anything.

@crazypharmd

I had a patient with crabs come in for treatment and he told me he was sleeping with his roommate's cat and that's where he got it from. He quickly added that he was not having sex with the cat but the cat was sleeping in his bed.

Stephen Riley

Another time when she started as a counter assistant she encountered a gentleman who sounded like he wanted something for cramps for his partner and rubbed around his stomach area when describing it. She couldn't understand why he was confused when she offered him Feminax. It was only when the pharmacist hurriedly came out it became apparent the gentleman had said crabs.

@PharMag_Richard

I was working as a pharmacist in one of the less salubrious parts of Portsmouth:

Customer: Have you got anything for crabs?

Assistant: Thousand Island dressing?

Sian Roberts

A woman asked to see me in private. We did not have any consultation rooms back then. We went into the manager's office. She asked me if I would check her for lice as she had nobody to ask! I was not keen, but decided to be nice. It had been a boring day and I was still a bit green! She then proceeded to unbuckle her belt! They were THOSE kind of lice! I actually screamed and scarpered then had to go back and apologise!!

Anon

This sounds like something from a teenage girl magazine but happened when I was in my mid-twenties. While I am always happy to turn up early for a locum appointment, I don't like staying late and like to get away on the dot. As we were just closing the pharmacy door at 5.30 (happy days!), a man slid around it. Cross that he had managed to get in, I stood my ground and asked him what he wanted. He mumbled something about doing rice and I thought he had mistaken us for the shop next door so I told him we didn't sell rice. In a slightly louder voice and in the hearing of all the staff, he said "I wanted something for pubic lice". That taught me a bit of a lesson.

John D'Arcy

Not long after qualifying, I worked as a locum in a pharmacy in Central London. It had a sound OTC business, and whilst I had an in-depth knowledge of the ins and outs of the dispensing part of the business I was less than knowledgeable about the OTC component of the business, and in particular, the brand names of products. One morning a rather well dressed and very well spoken woman entered the pharmacy and requested a packet of "Joy Rides". This was a product unfamiliar to me but as I did not want to appear ignorant I decided to use my initiative. A name like "Joy Rides" must apply to condoms and to avoid any embarrassment I removed the condom drawer from the rack and held it in front of her. Whilst I could not see the "Joy Rides" in amongst the selection of "Bareback", "French Delight" and "Ticklers" I felt sure she would be able to locate them. Instead, her face frowned up and she looked at me sternly. "They are travel sickness tablets", she said.

Anon

Just been told by my wife that during a respiratory MUR with an elderly gentleman, she was informed that he's going back to his GP in January for a blow job! She said I'm sure you'll feel better afterwards. It's amazing what you can get on the NHS these days!!

Joanne Myatt

I once had a lady bring in a sample for a pregnancy test in her husband's butty box (and it was half full!)

JonF

Or a yoghurt pot(with yoghurt still around the rim...yes this has happened!!!) covered in a bit of cling film!!!!

Nik

Once a staff member scanned a brown bottle with a barcode on, not realising until the lady told him, that it contained her urine sample.

Pharmanaut

We had one in a milk jug in a carrier bag. Young female customer did not warn us. Rule 1: always carry the pregnancy test sample upright as handed to you by the customer.

@mrdispenser

Just refused to accept a urine sample as surgery is shut. Lady must have thought I was taking the piss or not as the case may be...

We once had a full sample bottle posted through the letter box with a note asking us to take it to GP. Found it on a Monday AM!

El-loco

Story told to me by a dispenser some years ago - she swore it was true and I never had cause not to believe her. (If she reads this she'll know who she is!) They had as customers a young couple trying unsuccessfully for a child with the woman on fertility treatment. Every month her husband brought in her urine sample for a pregnancy test and every month it was negative - and on getting the result he always looked devastated. One month he brought in the sample and the result was the same - negative. Now in those days the tests could not detect pregnancy as early as today's can so thinking that the result might have been positive if the sample had been taken a day or two later and in an attempt to show sympathy the dispenser said "I think you might have come too early". She said he went red as a beetroot and replied that he couldn't help it.

Canadian Pharmacy

Canadian Pharmacists get into some crazy adventures.

Zhuyin (Sarah) Zhao

I once delivered a patient's controlled medications after she called us in a panic saying that she wouldn't be able to make it before closing. This wouldn't be so out of the ordinary except she lived in a very sketchy area of the city and I delivered her medications in my backpack on my bike. I also had to wait for her at a street corner and since she didn't show up for a while, tried to be very incognito while cars rolled by, with drivers suspiciously eyeing me. She never did show up but sent her underage child instead. I never thought I would be handing a bag of controlled substances to an underage child on a street corner on my bike as part of my job. It was quite the experience.

Mike Laevens

We had a guy admitted with alcoholic liver disease with the worst ascites I have ever witnessed. We recently hired three new pharmacist grads so I thought it would be a good teaching opportunity to show them. Well this guy also had the worst scrotal oedema I've seen and he was quite proud of it and was keen on showing them. Their reactions were great and it was a great introduction to hospital practice.

Anon

I now work in a medical clinic doing medication management and chronic disease management and certainly the most shocking thing that I have ever had happen in my career occurred recently. I guess because I use the same rooms as the physicians, patients think of me on the same level as a physician and it's not unusual for them to pull up their shorts or pull down their pants to show me a rash but a gentlemen actually brought in a sample of his ejaculate fluid (on a paper towel in a zip-loc bag) to ask if the brown streaking was blood!! I referred him to book an appointment with the physician to discuss that further (the doctor guessed that the blood was present as his masturbation was probably too vigorous), the man is 73 years old! I was so proud of myself for maintaining my composure. The reason I became a pharmacist and not a doctor was to avoid that kind of thing!

Andrea

Today was interesting... I showed a man how to give his cat Lantus and I helped a lady pick out a bottle and nipples for baby pigs!

Hugo Yeung

I had a homeless man in once a week asking for a new insulin pen because he'd get drunk and lose it. He'd be like:

"Hugo. I losht it. Get me a new pehn."

"Where is it?"

"I don't know! The ambulansh took it".

A real mess. He'd come in reeking of urine and stale beer. I don't take his BG because I can do a reading with the ketone smell. I even had a Febreeze bottle ready.

Well, one day, he stumbles in and we're talking the usual homeless talk and he tells me that his pants are falling off. Asks me if I could help him. I tell him Hell no, what kind of sick trick... Well, it turns out he was drunk and honest (his pants were loose because it had no buttons). So I, being in a particularly sick mood, grabbed a role of duct tape. I usually try to stay way behind the counter. That day, he smelled worse than a piss soaked bathroom floor at a bar. He lifts his shirt and I'm gagging.

This is at 11 am. I slap on the tape right where his hairy belly and pants meet. Push it in real good, and I pull hard and tight to get a good wrap all the way. Like it's ghetto Christmas and this guy is the worst present of all time. I proceeded to circle him four or five times wrapping duct tape around his rancid belly. He thanks me. Anyway, I spray some Febreeze and I'm looking at this guy with the duct tape belt, trying not to giggle. I get back to work and my tech goes "So, you're a pharmacist AND a tailor".

Emily Li

When I worked at the Glenrose I was visiting a patient to teach her how to use her multiple inhalers, and ended up, helping her change her sweater, put on her stockings, clean her

171

nightstand, change the water in her vase, and find her lipstick. Oh, and I was almost forced to eat a digestive cookie that looked like it had been sat on. 45 minutes later, she was too tired to learn how to use an Aerochamber, so I had to come back after naptime…I think this is proof that pharmacists are pretty much the nicest people out there – that, or we're just doormats.

Darren Pasay

I have fed a cat for a patient/neighbor who was in hospital.

Checked lotto numbers (many times).

Delivered mail, parcels and rent cheques.

Shredded credit card statements.

Picked up a bottle of rum (pre-ordered from the vendors) for a LTC resident.

Filled morphine bags for a dog.

Euthanized a fish.

Over The Counter

Pharmanaut

When asking for a medicinal product always get instantly annoyed when the person on the counter tries to make sure that it is not going to harm you, and that you know how to get the best from it. The more idiosyncratic your reaction the more points you score to boost your ego. Remember, extra points if for extra sarcasm, interruptions etc. Bonus points if you make the assistant want a career change. Maximum ego points if you suffer iatrogenic illness for not listening.

"Can't you just hurry up, I don't have time for all these questions?"

Make up the name of an old fashioned remedy, go in and ask them to order it. For example, Mr Spock's Alien Cure.

Always wink when you ask for a box of aspirins. It makes for a nice surprise when you open the bag when you get home.

Anything that says 'Natural' on it must be good for you.

Anything with maximum strength advertised on television is always better than what the pharmacist recommends.

Nik

Come into the pharmacy with a chesty cough and ask to speak to the pharmacist. When s/he asks you if you've tried anything for it, reply, "Yeah, I've borrowed some of my wife's antibiotics but they ain't touched it."

Run into the pharmacy 5 minutes before closing, holding a voucher for 20% off Nicorette gum 4mg. Watch the counter assistants go into the back trying to look for any remaining stock. Tell them to hurry up because Strictly come Dancing will start soon.

Demand an emergency supply of paracetamol as you have none left because you gave them to all your friends and family. When told about purchasing them over the counter, refuse to hand over money and tell the pharmacist to hurry up.

Customers: Help yourself to the medicines in the cupboards; you know the ones that have the notice "SUPERVISED SALE ONLY - PLEASE ASK FOR ASSISTANCE". You don't need any help of course, you just need to pick up your usual co-codamol and kaolin and morphine. Don't bother hassling us.

Go up to the counter and ask to see the pharmacist whilst 5 people are waiting for their meds - when s/he comes out start an in-depth discussion about the pros and cons of using echinacea for cold relief, and whether you should be using Bach flower remedies instead, because the witch doctor next door said so.

Go to the counter and ask to see the pharmacist. Complain about the wrong price of the shampoo you just bought. Once you see the pharmacist begin to get irritated, start shouting out loudly for a refund, complain about the ineptitude of counter staff and promise never to come back in the shop again.

Lilleymon

When the assistant asks you if you are taking any medication, say "yes". When they ask you what it is, say "It's white".

Weenoldo

One of our staff members recently took a stand against a regular co-codamol buyer:

Patient: Packet of co-codamol please.

Assistant: Can I just check what it's for?

Patient: Oh I've got a really sore back.

Assistant: It's just because you've been in for a box a few times in the last couple of weeks so I can't sell it to you.

Patient: Oh, ok. Well can I get a box for my friend? She has a really sore back.

Grumpyoldwoman

I hate it when someone asks for 'advice' on something ... then, having gone through it all, they say "Well, I had [whatever] last time & it seemed to work, I'll have that again please".

"I didn't want to bother the doctor because he's so busy, I thought I'd ask you".

Patient: "I need some eyedrops."

Assistant: "What do you need them for?"

Patient: "My wife's eyes".

Veteran Locum

1) Male customers who elect to wait and then stand with their hands in their pockets jingling their loose change and keys around their external genitalia; I do in fact ask myself in these cases whether it is some form of implied challenge, which will be achieved first, the prescription in a bag or orgasm?

2) People who ask your advice on what medicine to take. So you recommend X. They then say either "but I've got some of that at home" or " but someone told me to take..."

Stressed

"It's none of your business what medication I'm on, you're not a doctor!"

My personal favourite reply to "What medicines are you currently taking"... You know...those small white tablets".

"It's ok, my doctor knows" The GMC would be very busy if all these GPs were really turning a blind eye to codeine addiction!

Honest

"What have you got for...? I've tried everything already".

Dizzyb23

LOL (aka Little Old Lady) very politely throws an empty box and bottle of Benylin dry cough med at me and says "Refill me luv"!!!! I do the WWHAM stuff and she basically ignores me completely and demands the "refill"..... Her cough is clearly chesty, she's had it months and is not feeling well plus she's on loads of other meds but not from us as she usually goes to Boots. My Pharmacist is doing an MUR of course so I can't get help. Our conversation gets more and more heated (on her part not mine). I then tell her I'm not selling her the cough med, she looks at me as though I'm made of c*** and tells me she'll go get it from Boots as they are a much better chemist.

Sir Dispensalot

Feel free to forget about the list of existing prescription medicines you already take when buying OTC medication - especially the ones which have potentially life-threatening interactions, the pills you buy can't possibly harm you, after all. Once in hospital, allow any close family member or hospital doctor to telephone and tear strips off your pharmacist.

Get exceedingly angry when the pharmacist won't sell you the 4 boxes of Sudafed/Nytol/Night Nurse you desperately need to store in your kitchen cupboard 'just in case'. Get even madder when he won't sell any more boxes to the person you came into the shop with.

Feel free to get angry when the pharmacist won't just sell you Viagra under the counter without prescription, after all they don't care about getting struck off, do they?

Phone

Weenoldo

Phone up the pharmacy at 1pm on a Saturday (bang on closing time) and say "my brother's on his way down with a script, he's in 'Placeabout4milesaway', can you hold on til he gets there?" When I refuse, shout about how he really needs this medication and he'll end up in hospital without it. To which, of course, I reply...all together now..."then why did he leave it until he had none left and it was 1pm on a Saturday?"

@AmberRaeParks

My phone just autocorrected "maybe" to "NSAID".

Jo McMillan

If the phone rings before opening time, I personally prefer "no, I'm just the cleaner, ducks!"

Defblade

Never answer the phone within 5 minutes of closing (and certainly not within 2 or 3 minutes). It's ALWAYS this. Exception is if you're in a very rural pharmacy and there might genuinely be trouble getting to the next supermarket pharmacy that's open till 8/9/12 at night.

Pharmanaut

Phone the pharmacy at closing time asking for a quote on anti-malarials for a party of 10 ranging from adult to children of all different ages. Then say it's cheaper at xyz pharmacy.

Weenoldo

And a special mention to our nursing homes: If you're phoning up the pharmacy because you don't seem to have an item for a certain patient, never actually look to see if you have the item first. Best to make sure the pharmacy has searched every nook and cranny of their shop first before realising it was in your medication trolley all along.

Phone up to order your repeat prescription, and when asked what your name is, say "Mrs Smith". You know, that one Mrs Smith?

kl06229

Guy phones up on a Saturday and asks us to order his prescription for Quinine sulphate, "I've not ran out but I want it to be ready for me by Monday morning". He's told in the most polite way possible that this isn't possible but pharmacist helpfully suggests if he's got a reason for needing it so soon he should give the doctor a quick ring first thing on Monday. The pharmacist is told to "go to hell!"

Receive a phone call, person asking "What time does Greggs the bakers nearby close?"

@PharmacyProblems

I love when people call and when we answer they're on the line yelling at their families.

No really, please continue your phone conversation while I ask you a few questions.

181

Miscellaneous

Patient came in and said to me that she had collected her prescription from a different pharmacy. There was a note on her script saying that the locum wanted a word. She asked me what he wanted a word about…

John D'Arcy

During the early 90s there was much debate and discussion about pharmacy's future role and therefore a major focus on whether there was indeed any future for community pharmacy. The PJ at the time was filled with letters on the subject and the standard topic for meetings of RPS branches, LPCs and so on was "Is there a Future for Community Pharmacy?" I was invited to speak at such a meeting in Barnsley.

I stood up to speak and put the titles slide up. Just as I was about to start, a guy at the back began waving his hand excitedly and shouting "excuse me".

"Can I help?" I asked.

"Is it okay if I ask a question?" he said.

"Of course it is, although I must say that it is most unusual to ask a question before I have actually said anything" was my reply.

"I'm just looking at the title of your presentation – Is there a future for community pharmacy?" he said, "I am assuming the answer is yes, because if it is 'no' I will get my coat and leave now."

@sjhoward [Dr]

I prescribed Milk of Magnesia to a patient when I worked at the hospital. I came back the next day and a nurse had written on the Kardex: 'Milk of magnesia not available. Milk of cow given instead.

@zams123

On a normal day at work, an 80-year old woman brought her script in. We did not have some of her medicines in stock (it was rare expensive stock). I informed her of this and she kicked off at me in front of a shop full of people. I remained calm and told her the stock would be available in the afternoon, she could come back or get someone else to pick it up for her or we could deliver the next morning. This was not good enough for her and she was extremely rude, she wanted her meds there and then. I gave her script back which she snatched off me and took somewhere else....I quite gladly wished I also should have told her not to come back again! Today, the same woman swallowed a Canesten pessary by mistake..! And had the guts to tell me and ask me for advice... How she managed to swallow that big pessary?

Darshana Thaker

I had a lady come up to me with the strongest Jamaican accent asking me whether I had frankincense and Mer. I thought I hadn't heard her correctly so asked her again and she raised her voice and repeated. Everyone in the dispensary was laughing their heads off and I was trying to keep a straight face. I explained that we didn't and she blew into a fit saying we should have it and how she finds it impossible to believe we haven't.

Monica Elaine

Patient: What time do you close today?

Me: 6pm

Patient: So I have to come before 6?

Sarah L

How silly of me to expect you to know your surgery is closed on a Saturday, they've only been doing that for the last 8 years!

@josephbush

I was once asked by a patient collecting two creams, which one went on her labia majora and which on her labia minora. Did not have a clue and she didn't use the scientific names either.

Jauna

Most unique Sudafed story to date: a woman came in yesterday saying she needed Sudafed 24 hour for her dog. She said her dog has the same sinus problems that she does and the dog has sinus headaches like her too. I don't know about you, but my dog never complains of headaches. Poor dog!

Zoggite

I gave out some metronidazole 400mg tabs today; as I warned the patient not to consume alcohol whilst taking these, he replied "am I OK with cannabis, though?"

Al Jones

Lady walks in complaining of on-going breathing difficulties. She was recently diagnosed with mild asthma and was prescribed salbutamol prn. She came into the pharmacy for her repeat inhaler and said that it wasn't working, at which point the pharmacist sat her down in the consultation room and ran through some basic questions. Suspecting a technique problem, they asked her to demonstrate using it. She replied that since she used it for her cat allergy, it obviously wouldn't work without her cat around. Slightly confused, the pharmacist humoured her and asked her to pretend a nearby cushion was the cat. She promptly doused the cushion in salbutamol.

Lisa Butler

A woman came in and asked if we sold eggs once and a gentleman got very angry when he realised we didn't have a post box in store. Also, one customer got so angry at the price of a prescription charge that the pharmacist offered to charge him the actual price; it was for something like Lyrica.

@Alkemist1912

Somebody once asked me for the morning before pill. You couldn't make it up.

@Dr_L_78

A Latvian patient asked me for the anti-baby pill on Friday. I also had a bizarre consultation with a young man who had scrotal irritation but kept referring to his ball sack in all seriousness.

Abs

Why every pharmacist should take first aid training seriously. I had gone through my pharmacy career doing the occasional provision of an inhaler helping someone who'd fainted or had an epileptic seizure but nothing could have prepared me for an elderly lady who came in to the pharmacy and collapsed. I went over to her and did the usual checks and realised she wasn't breathing and my mind went blank. Fortunately I recovered and gave her CPR (mouth to mouth included). Even though she had slipped away I continued till the paramedics arrived.

One by one the other customers left the pharmacy save for one elderly lady who sat on a chair patiently waiting. Once I had finished talking to the paramedics my mind was on the girls in the shop who were all pretty shaken. I was too but I had to keep my cool. Anyway, the elderly lady casually sidestepped the woman's body and handed over her prescription. I told her she would have to wait because I was in no condition to dispense her prescription safely and that we had to deal with the situation at hand she went off in a huff. 20 minutes later whilst I was still trying to sort things out I got a phone call from our friendly PCT head of pharmacy asking why we found it appropriate to close the pharmacy without informing him just because we had some 'sort of bereavement'. That was the straw that broke the camel's back, I burst in to tears and screamed 'There's a dead body on the floor!' he muttered I'm ever so sorry and put down the phone. Apparently, the woman was unimpressed that I had refused to dispense her PPI and rang the PCT to complain!

@AdamPlum

I was at the usual place of work and on my own as my full timer was out delivering. A family of Japanese tourists came in and walked up to the counter. The man had a hand-held Psion type device which had a lot of Japanese characters on it and then a single English word.. "cream".

He then pointed to another woman and her face and pointed to the screen which read "itchy". I nodded and went over to where I felt I would have a cream that would be suitable. I then heard a "beep beep" and dismissed it. I tried to convey what the cream was for and then pointed at the woman's face. And another "beep beep". Ignored it.

Walked over to the counter, used the till and heard another "beep beep" ... As I handed over the change, the man bowed and held out his hand with the money in it for longer than anticipated. I heard a "beep beep" and then a woman lent forward with a camcorder in her hand. She had been filming the whole consultation without me even realising.....I was on my own version of "You've been Framed" for a Japanese family's holiday video. 'For years to come, I will be the butt of a Japanese family's holiday video anecdote'.

@fuzzdammit

Male topless stripper coming in and buying Quinoderm as his skin is too greasy. He had a part as an extra in Casualty apparently.

kl06229

Old man comes in to ask the pharmacist about his ointment. He doesn't know which one, just some ointment. "I think it's called oxybutynin ointment" I skim through his PMR and see oxybutynin tablets and hydrocortisone ointment. You see where this is going don't you? I ask him if maybe he's confused the names, then he calls the dispenser over because "this guy doesn't know what he's talking about".

There was the patient with a script for 500ml benzyl benzoate. This was a thick, white liquid dispensed in those days in large fluted amber bottles, with the directions "To apply to the affected part". I dispensed this to the patient – a large bucolic gentleman in his 50s – with my usual cheery manner. Two days later he returned, and beckoned me over. "Look 'ere" he said, "You remember that stuff you gave me?" I nodded. "Well, do you know it was going to burn...you know, me privates!" I began to recall that benzyl benzoate was a scabicide – one no longer used owing to its irritant properties.

"Ahh..." I began, but he butted in and leaned towards me. "Yes you did – you were laughing. You're laughing now!" I realised that a nervous – and in the circumstances – hazardous grin had crept across my face. "No, I'm not!" I protested. I can only assume that my obvious ignorance was transmitted to him, as he seemed to back down. "Well" he said, "I'm still itching. What should I do?" To this day I am uncertain as to whether I was also ignorant of the fact that the pruritus of scabies can persist some weeks after eradication, or just feeling vengeful since my professionalism had been challenged, but I looked him square in the eye and said "Keep applying until the itching stops!"

@Redheadedpharmacist

This exchange happened between a customer and a pharmacy manager I was working with just last week at work:

Customer: "Hey, my husband finally got that colonoscopy."

Pharmacy manager: "Really?"

Customer: "Yeah, and guess what? They found three things!"

Pharmacy manager: (Face turns really serious) "Oh no!"

But before the pharmacy manager could say anything else....

Customer: "Yeah, they found two remotes and that shoe of mine that was missing."

Random thoughts of mine

Why do pharmacies keep back pain products on the bottom shelf?

People only want to talk to me once I start sucking a boiled sweet.

Whoever says that drugs are not dangerous has clearly never been hit in the face with a BNF.

During Euro 2012, I heard two patients say that 'he's too slow' in the pharmacy. I got upset until I realised that they were talking about Frank Lampard.

Please step away from the counter once you have handed your script in, otherwise you will get asked more than once if you are being served!

Life is like an AAH box. You never know which generic you're going to get.

Bored of patient satisfaction surveys? Save time by singing to patients "If you're happy and you know it, clap your hands". You get quantifiable data.

I like it when a patient has the same birthday as me.

That moment when a patient hands in a 6 page prescription & you look to your colleague & say, "I think we're going to need a bigger basket!"

Today, I will go into McDonalds, order 6 happy meals and tell them that I have a taxi waiting and see if they give a crap.

Generally, I'm a 'tube' man but if someone needs a label on the tube of toothpaste to tell them to brush twice daily then there is a bigger problem to deal with.

When a patient sees me count the number of tablets in a split dispensed box, it does nothing to dismiss the myth that I just count tablets.

Bored? Shove as many tablets as possible into the smallest box possible. Sit on it until it closes and then hand to pharmacist to check.

Technician gave me a script to check today and told me to just glance at it as it was right. Thanks for the heads-up.

Dear GPs, if and this is a really big if, you are really telling patients to buy co-codamol or Nytol etc. over the counter, please give them a note. Thanks.

Addict just sent a text to the shop landline saying that he has just got out of court and is on his way.

Today, an 18-year old patient had to confirm with her friends that September was the 9th month when dating her prescription. She's off to university.

There is always that one dispensing label that disappears during the day like magic. Its normally found stuck on your ass when you get home.

The I before E except after C rule does not apply when putting away the dispensary order.

Playing I-Spy with staff in dispensary is a great way to boost staff morale and help them remember drugs. Waiting times may increase though.

Apparently asking two guys standing at the counter if they are together is inappropriate and I'm stupid.

Patient asks for Sudafed. Assistant asks if she is on any blood pressure tablets. Patient replies, "Just because I'm fat, it doesn't mean I have high BP!"

My brother is so happy. Tears of joy. Did he get his A Level results today? No. Did he finally get his Orlistat prescription dispensed? Yes

My dad was always a firm believer of saying no to drugs. That's one reason he got fired from the pharmacy.

Patient asked for an emergency supply this morning as they no longer had their FP10 because their dog ate it!

Summer student got told off this morning for daring to say 'good morning' to a patient who quite clearly was not having a good morning!

Slightly surreal sight when the patient wanted to shake the erythromycin suspension so we let him. Audience participation aids compliance. Although we have now had to enroll him on a dispensing course now as per regulations.

Surgery shut again for training this afternoon. I've yet to see the fruits of its labour! Let me do the training!

If you sign all prescriptions in the blue box, you may be institutionalised.

The people that say 'Well, it's a free country, aint it!' are probably the ones that don't pay for their prescriptions.

One of Team Menopause today said that they feel cold. Has hell frozen over?

If you turn up to collect an owing without your owing slip, then be prepared for disapproving looks & a chat with our technician/interrogator.

Dear manufacturers, when naming a new drug, please choose a name that I can spell and pronounce & won't automatically give me 50 points in Scrabble!

I checked a prescription today which had a near miss on it. I told the dispenser who genuinely said "Ooh, it's a good job you checked' with no hint of irony.

Dear drug manufacturers, please make tablets in packs of 31 to avoid me getting shouted at. Thank you.

Hey, I just met you and this is crazy. You are on a new diabetes tablet, so can I call you maybe? #NMS

My methadone brings all the boys to the yard and they're like "Hurry up, I've got a taxi waiting.

Epilogue

If you have enjoyed this book as much as I have enjoyed writing it, then please let me know via mrdispenser@hotmail.co.uk. If there is enough interest, then I will write and compile another book. If you have a funny story about pharmacy, please share it.

I will leave you with this anecdote from @drwalker_rph:

Five years after I left dispensing pharmacy I ran into one of my former patients. When I was practicing pharmacy I probably saw him several times a month at the pharmacy. I had not seen him for over 5 years and happened to run into him when I was in the store shopping. He explained he has Alzheimer's dementia and struggles with his memory even forgetting the names of people he sees every day. But I was pleased when he told me he always remembered my name as his former pharmacist...

Glossary

AAH: A wholesaler.

Alliance: Another wholesaler.

Blacklisted: The NHS only allows doctors to prescribe certain products. The ones that are not allowed are on the Black List.

Broken Bulk: Medicines come in a variety of pack sizes. Some may come in a 100 pack. If you get a prescription for only 20 and then never see another prescription, the medicine goes out of date. If you claim Broken Bulk, the first time you dispense, and then you do not lose out.

CD: Controlled Drug.

ETP: Electronic Transfer of Prescriptions.

Lipotrim: Weight loss service offered by pharmacies. Others are available.

MDS: Monitored dosage tray. Also known as nomad or Venalink. Tablets are popped out and placed in weekly trays.

Medicines Use Review: Another service in which the pharmacist goes through each medication with the patient to see if they are getting the most of out of them.

Methameasure: A machine that measures out the correct dose of methadone for a patient.

NCSO: No Cheaper Stock Obtainable. We get reimbursed a set price for what we dispense. Sometimes that product is out of stock and if a drug is granted NCSO status by the Department of

Health, then we can temporarily supply a more expensive product and get reimbursed for it.

Near miss log: A record of the accuracy mistakes that a pharmacist/accredited checking technician have found that have not reached the patient.

New Medicines Service: If a patient has a newly prescribed medicine for either high blood pressure, Type 2 diabetes, asthma/COPD or blood thinning, then they are eligible for this service.

NPA: National Pharmacy Association.

NWOS: North West Ostomy Supplies: A company that supplies dressings and other products.

Proscript: A computer program used to generate labels. Others are available.

QDS: Four times daily.

SOP: Standard Operating Procedure. The set way of doing most things in the pharmacy.

Made in the USA
Lexington, KY
15 September 2014